Praise for

Heart of the Matter

"*Working with Lynn to raise awareness about cardiac arrest has given me a personal way to give back, much like my mother did for breast cancer and addiction. As* Heart of the Matter *shows, there's still so much work to be done—and **this book empowers every reader** to be part of the solution to save lives.*

*As a fellow survivor, **I'm grateful to Lynn** for sharing her experiences in* Heart of the Matter—*it reminded me we're never truly alone after surviving.*"

–**Susan Ford Bales,** Cardiac Arrest Survivor and Daughter of the 38th President of the United States, Gerald R. Ford and First Lady Betty Ford

"*Though I don't remember most of the calls I've gone on as a firefighter, **I will never forget Valentine's Day 2007.** The quick actions of her colleagues and the Emergency Medicine applied on scene brought Lynn back to life, but what has been most remarkable about that day is the life Lynn gave back in response to it. The story of her journey back from cardiac arrest is **remarkable, inspiring and something well worth reading** . . .*"

–**Ryan Sutter,** Firefighter and Star of ABC's hit reality series *The Bachelorette*

"*Lynn Blake's heart is like a Notre Dame football helmet at the end of the season: chipped and wounded, yet still gold. If you are wondering what resilience looks like, **read this book.**"

–**Devon O'Neil,** Acclaimed Freelance Journalist and Author of *The Way Out*

"*An incredibly inspiring memoir that highlights extraordinary ways Lynn's paid it forward. The ideas, commitment, and impact are amazing. **I hope to follow in even a few of the ways Lynn has.**"

–**Robert Kalmowitz,** Cardiac Arrest Survivor

"*Lynn's story is a rare gift—equal parts heart-stopping and heart-opening.* Heart of the Matter *doesn't just chronicle survival; it illuminates purpose,* resilience, and the quiet ways we find our way back to ourselves. I'm **grateful she had the courage to write it—and even more grateful we get to read it.**"

−**J. Brooks,** Founder & CEO, GlassView

"Lynn Blake's work **moved me to my core.** Her story of surviving sudden cardiac arrest is so much more than a story of survival—it's a story of awakening. With raw honesty, grace, and depth, she invites us into the most vulnerable parts of her journey and shows us what it means to alchemize pain into purpose. It's a powerful reminder of what it means to really live."

−**Kate Leatherby,** Paramedic

"What a fantastic read! Powerful and inspiring, this book is rich with details—capturing the challenges and triumphs of recovery, medical procedures, emotional turmoil, and personal growth. Lynn's honesty and openness make this journey incredibly engaging. **Thank you for sharing such an inspirational and heartfelt story.**"

−**Alan Owen,** Cardiac Arrest Survivor

"Deeply engaging and profoundly personal, Lynn's work opens a path for others to explore the eternal in their own lives. I wholeheartedly applaud her mission to bring encouragement and hope to others. I am truly excited to witness the **transformative impact this book will have on so many lives!**"

−**Craig Smith,** Pastor of The Vail Church

"Part educational, part inspirational, and part intimate. An enthralling memoir that invites readers into an intimate journey of resilience and hope. With vivid storytelling and a relatable narrative, this book offers a powerful, inspiring message for anyone facing adversity. A must-read for those who find strength in stories of triumph over life's challenges. **Every reader will walk away with something.**"

−**Alexia B.,** Reader

"A beautifully crafted story of **intense, vivid moments** with dark clouds transformed into radiant silver linings."

−**Rachel W.,** Reader

Heart of the Matter

How My Near-Death Experiences
Led Me to Save Lives and Souls

Heart of the Matter

Lynn Blake

For permission requests, write to:
Heart Hope, PO Box 9152, Avon, CO 81620 ID: 20101219885
Email: requests@hearthope.org

Heart Hope, a registered nonprofit, dedicates a portion of the proceeds from
Heart of the Matter to supporting charitable organizations that save lives and
souls. EIN: 27-2377254
HeartHope.org

ISBN (paperback): 979-8-9993855-0-5
ISBN (hardcover): 979-8-9993855-1-2
ISBN (ebook): 979-8-9993855-2-9
ISBN (audio): 979-8-9993855-3-6

Book design and production by www.AuthorSuccess.com

For my fellow survivors, and for the lives
and souls this book will help save.

FREE Added Bonus for Download

Visit HeartHope.org to download your free copy of the bonus material: *The Big Questions: Answers from the Perspective of a Survivor* found at the end of *Heart of the Matter.*

Reader Advisory: The added bonus is not for everyone. Only read it if you're open to exploring big questions—and extreme possibilities. After surviving cardiac arrest, I found myself wrestling with life's greatest mysteries:

- **What's our purpose and time to live?**
- **Does God exist?**
- **What happens when we die?**
- **How do we find peace with the unknowns of life?**

These questions consumed me in a fierce pursuit of answers. I spent years searching, reading, reflecting, and confronting both science and religion. What emerged wasn't certainty, but a deeper connection to life, death, purpose, and ultimate peace.

Here's the invitation: If you're curious, if you're questioning, if you're ready to consider that something greater might be in control of life, this is for you!

FREE LIFESAVING Resources

Visit SaveMoreLives.org

Whether you're a survivor, want to know how to save a life, or simply someone who cares, these tools are designed to support your efforts.

Learn CPR in Minutes
Watch our **quick CPR: Call–Pump–Restart** video and learn the essential steps to respond to cardiac arrest.

Purchase a Lifesaving Defibrillator/AED
The majority of cardiac arrests occur in the home–make sure your family is protected today!

Start a Fundraiser for a Lifesaving Defibrillator/AED
Equip the places you visit. Rally your friends, neighbors, or workplace to raise funds for a defibrillator in your community.

Shop Thoughtful Gifts for Survivors and Heros
Comfort someone impacted by cardiac arrest, or acknowledge the people who helped save a life.

Share Your Story or Honor a Loved One
Your story matters! Connect and inspire others by sharing your experiences with cardiac arrest.

Support the Mission
Make a donation to help support projects and organizations that help save lives and inspire hope for the heart.

HeartHope.org

Contents

Author's Note   xiii

Part 1 The Main Event
1   The Proposal and the Path Ahead   3
2   Heartbeats of a New Life   9
3   On the Edge of Life   14
4   In Sickness and in Health   18
5   Miracles in the Storm   24
6   Uncertain Future   30
7   Cognitive Fog   35
8   When Heaven Is Quiet   40
9   The Scar on My Chest   45
10   Four Life-Changing Words   49
11   A Screen of False Promises   54
12   Much Needed Change   64
13   Am I The Only One Questioning?   71
14   The Two Most Pivotal Gifts   76

Part 2 Life After Cardiac Arrest
15   Hidden Connections   83
16   Ascending From the Valley   87
17   Mountain of Purpose   93
18   Building a Heart-Driven Movement   102
19   No Data, No Dollars   109
20   Signs From Above   114
21   Lightening the Load   123
22   The Final Stretch   126
23   The First Real Baby   137
24   One Fall and Call Away   141
25   Summoning the Courage   145
26   There's Always an Obstacle Ahead   148
27   Leaving My Baby Behind   153

28 Long Days, Fast Years &   158
       Instructions for Creating A "Days of Your Life" Jar
29 The One I Waited For   165
30 Life is Never Boring   170
31 It All Ends the Same Way   179

Conclusion   187
17 Steps to Reduce Anxiety and Increase Heart Hope   191

References   193
Acknowledgements   194
Bonus Material: The Big Questions   197

Author's Note

Every time I tell the story of surviving cardiac arrest, I hesitate to reveal the deeper layers. Life has shaped me into an introvert—a seeker of quiet corners, a soul most at peace in solitude. Though I've always been contemplative, I've learned that inwardness doesn't mean avoiding visibility altogether. Putting myself out there has never been natural, but sometimes, stepping into the spotlight becomes a form of advocacy and healing. When the cause is deeply personal and the stakes are real, you find courage you didn't know you had. I've often scribbled my thoughts in pencil, ready to erase them at any moment, afraid of the permanence of my words. Sharing these experiences with you in legible ink is as terrifying as it is cathartic.

When I survived at the age of 27 in 2007, I was desperate to understand what had happened—not just medically, but emotionally, spiritually, and practically. Understanding the impact of this bewildering incident on my life was crucial for me to progress.

I scoured bookshelves, looking for stories like mine. I found almost none. Even now, they're rare. The reasons are heartbreakingly simple. First, few people survive cardiac arrest and live to tell about it. For those who do, recovery takes time—for physical healing, and most importantly, the freedom to process it all. Finally, it requires extraordinary strength to overcome the invisible wounds that remain: the anxiety, the procedures, the lingering awareness that life can end in a heartbeat. To share it is to relive it.

Nearly two decades later, I've walked a long path of self-discovery. I've faced my mortality, wrestled with purpose, and adjusted to life with an implanted pacemaker defibrillator. Guided by faith and a growing conviction, I turned my ordeals into advocacy—founding a nonprofit and championing legislation to raise awareness about cardiac arrest.

But for years, I kept parts of myself hidden—trapped by silence, fear of judgment, and the pressure to appear perfect. I buried struggles with body image, personal habits, emotional wounds, and even committing a criminal offense behind a polished surface. Eventually, my commitment and passions pushed me to step forward, to share what I had kept locked away, and to open a door for others seeking healing and hope.

At the end of each chapter in Part 2, you'll find a practical "Step to Reduce Anxiety and Increase Heart Hope"—simple, actionable ideas to help navigate life's uncertainties. One special practice, the "Days of Your Life" jar, invites you to treasure each day as the gift it truly is.

While I couldn't entirely separate my story from spiritual and religious perspectives, I attempted to limit their influence, hoping to connect with a broader audience. Still, I believe the considerations are too important to ignore. For those seeking deeper reflections on life's unknowns, an additional bonus, "The Big Questions" from the perspective of a survivor, is included.

Thank you for walking this trail with me. I hope it leaves you with more peace, less fear, and perhaps even the confidence to save a life.

With all my heart,

Lynn

PART 1

The Main Event

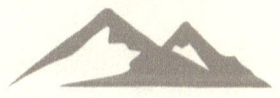

CHAPTER 1
The Proposal and the Path Ahead

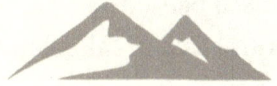

On an overcast July evening in 2006, three years after Matt and I first met, I felt something momentous brewing. Matt, ever thoughtful, had planned a dinner date at the Tennessee Pass Cookhouse, a rustic yurt near the Continental Divide. The location was approximately 40 minutes from where we lived in Vail, Colorado—a place known for its world-class skiing, luxury hotels, and gourmet dining. But this spot was nothing like that. Tucked deep in the mountains, this restaurant had no running water, just a round canvas structure with outhouses and a rugged charm. It was a scene where white tablecloths set beneath open skies and flickering lanterns are enough. It was the opposite of the fancy places in the resort villages we were accustomed to.

The details of the night reflected Matt's intent: he swapped his trusty, rusted Subaru for a borrowed Toyota Matrix from his Help-U-Sell Real Estate office, a subtle but meticulous touch that made me smile.

I wore a breezy green and blue sundress with hiking shoes on my feet and heels tucked in my pack—just in case we snapped a photo. The air hummed with anticipation. As we drove to the destination, Matt's excitement was infectious. He smiled softly, and I mirrored his restraint, holding back my suspicions to savor the moment he had so carefully orchestrated.

At the trailhead, I shrugged into my rain jacket, a defense against the lingering drizzle. We began a short walk toward a monument honoring the Tenth Mountain Division soldiers. Rain-kissed wildflowers lined the narrow path, their delicate fragrance mingling with the earthy scent of wet soil. The intimacy of the moment felt like a quiet prelude to something life-changing.

And then, as if earth itself paused to witness, Matt stopped. Nerves overtook him, and in a fumbling break from tradition, he stayed on both feet, pulling a small box from his pocket. The lid snapped open to reveal a radiant two-carat diamond ring, its facets catching the faint light of the peaking sun. With heartfelt honesty, Matt confessed his love and asked me to be his wife. My breath hitched—not just from the mountain air, but from the sincerity in Matt's eyes. He didn't prepare anything elaborate, but I heard everything I needed in his voice. He had chosen me, fully and without hesitation. It wasn't just a proposal; it was a promise that wherever life took us, we'd walk it together. The moment was simple and deeply real—more meaningful than any grand gesture I could've imagined.

My heart pounded in joy, echoing the rhythm of the moment. 'Yes!' I exclaimed, the word carrying all the certainty and excitement in my soul.

On cue, the clouds parted, bathing us in warm sunlight.

A lone deer darted across the path, as if the universe blessed our union. It felt surreal—like something out of a dream, yet it was real, marking the beginning of our new life.

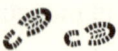

What I loved most about Matt wasn't just how effortlessly he crushed telemark turns down the most difficult runs or how handsome he was—though certainly noticed. It was the way I knew, from the very beginning, that we were meant to be.

His first glance said it all. There was goodness in him. Depth. Strength. Assured. A quiet confidence that didn't need to prove itself. He was the full package—athletic, intelligent, kind. Raised Irish Catholic and second-oldest out of four, Matt learned the value of commitment and dedication early. He watched his dad work long hours to make ends meet. That stuck with him. He knew life required effort and gave everything his all. He finished high school at the top of his class, earning titles like Most Likely to Succeed and Athlete of the Year before being recruited by Middlebury College for both hockey and baseball. And yet, he remained humble. He didn't chase attention—it found him.

We're both introverts. Not withdrawn, just wired to listen, notice, and invest deeply. Some of the quietest people form the strongest bonds. They notice what matters. That was us. Our deepest connection unfolded in motion—hiking switchbacks, riding a chairlift, lost in conversation—or silence. The quiet never felt empty. It felt like home.

For me, love lived in slight gestures. I noticed the ones left out, those who needed a little extra care. I didn't love loudly, but I loved with intention. A handmade card, a spontaneous bouquet of flowers, a note of encouragement. The connection itself mattered to me.

And that's the kind of love we shared. Steady. Grounded. Real. The kind that shows up when no one's watching. The kind that stays.

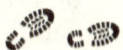

On the drive home, Matt showcased his extraordinary talent: identifying Grateful Dead shows by year and selecting the best set for any moment. He slipped in a cassette of their September 20, 1970, performance. As Jerry Garcia's voice crooned from *New Speedway Boogie* into *Brokedown Palace*, the lyrics confirmed everything we were feeling. We loved each other more than words could tell. . . .

We knew then that we'd listen to the river sing sweet songs to rock our souls during the first dance as husband and wife

When we shared the news with our families, their joy reflected ours. My mother, her voice full of emotion, gripped Matt's arm and said, "I've been praying for Lynn's husband since she was born. We couldn't be more pleased that it's you."

With our families' support, the planning began. My mom's insistence that we set a wedding date within six months gave us a nudge we needed, and soon, the dreamy white winter wedding took shape.

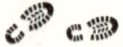

The details came together effortlessly. February felt like the perfect fit, capturing the snowy, magical atmosphere we'd imagined. It also doubled as a ski vacation for our guests. We chose the charming interfaith chapel for our ceremony and a grand timber-and-stone lodge for the reception, both nestled along Gore Creek—a trickling frozen stream lined with aspens and evergreens, flowing west through the heart of Vail, and the ski mountain rising in the background. It was the perfect setting.

Margaret, my older sister, graciously offered her wedding gown. When I tried it on, it fit perfectly with no alterations needed—simple, strapless, elegant. But at that moment, I couldn't help but be grateful that the biting words she'd once spoken were not prophetic.

Growing up, we shared a bathroom that connected our bedrooms. Mornings became a daily battleground, her slow, meticulous routines clashing with my impatience to get to school and see my friends.

"MARGARET!" I'd shout, pounding on her door. "It's time to GO! Your hair can dry on the way to school!"

The blow dryer was her only response. I'd kick the door in frustration, desperate to hurry her along. When she finally emerged, her words cut deeper than the wait.

"Lynn," she snapped, "you're so selfish that no one will ever marry you."

Although deserved, that comment haunted me long after it was made. I admired Margaret, which is why her words cut so deeply. Like all sisters, we knew exactly when to throw a sharp remark to claim a small victory. Yet beneath those fleeting battles, she was always in my corner. She had always been there for me and always would be. Beneath the tension, I still admired Margaret.

Margaret always seemed so perfect, a paragon of grace and maturity. She thrived in our structured household, her sense of style impeccable, her demeanor calm and composed. She was everything I wanted to be. Yet, I couldn't help but contrast myself with her. Where Margaret exuded polish, I embraced action. I was the wild child—the vinegar to her oil. I rolled down hills until my clothes were stained green, spun on tire swings until I was dizzy, and constantly pushed boundaries. While Margaret found joy in fashion and social graces, I sought adventure.

Despite our differences, I always wanted to emulate Margaret. Now, wearing her perfect wedding dress, I felt an unspoken bond between us—a connection rooted in our shared history and love.

One non-negotiable came from my mother: the ceremony had to be officiated by a pastor. Though Matt and I were raised in religious homes, we had long since drifted from our spiritual lives. Church was not a priority. We had become "ChrEasters"—those who attended church only on Christmas and Easter—but we respected my mother's wishes.

The family pastor at my parents' congregation, The Vail Church, agreed to officiate—on one condition: Matt and I had to attend premarital counseling, *and* it would be good if we attended on Sundays. I remember sitting in the car after our first session, engine off, both of us staring straight ahead.

"Did that feel weird to you?" I asked, finally breaking the silence

Matt let out a short laugh. "Not weird. Just . . . formal. Like, we were trying to give the right answers."

"I know. I kept thinking, *is this what we believe? Or what we think we're supposed to say?*"

He turned to look at me. "I mean, I do believe in something bigger. But I don't connect with church the way you're supposed to. It always felt like an obligation."

"Same," I said.

"We don't have to be perfectly aligned," he replied gently. "We just need to be honest. And respectful. I think that's what really matters."

In that moment, I realized we didn't have to perform belief—we just had to move forward in whatever way that looked like for us.

To our surprise, Pastor Craig's weekly sermons were relatable and authentic, resonating with both of us. A former professional athlete who had even spent time in Major League Baseball, Craig was a stark contrast to the stern priests of Matt's Catholic upbringing and the uninspiring preachers of my youth.

Amid the wedding preparations, a fresh opportunity presented itself. While skimming the *Vail Daily* classifieds, I spotted a job listing at the Vail Valley Partnership. Something about the ad called to me, so I clipped it out and pinned it to my corkboard—a declaration of intent for this new chapter of my life.

The interview went smoothly. My experience and enthusiasm seemed to impress Allison, the hiring manager. Days later, she called to offer me the job. I was thrilled but hesitant to start right away. With the wedding fast approaching, I worried about taking time off so soon after beginning. Thankfully, Allison understood, and we agreed on a start date of February 13—just in time for Valentine's Day.

CHAPTER 2
Heartbeats of a New Life

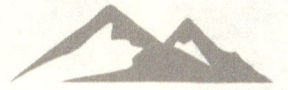

February arrived in a flurry of snow, blanketing the mountains as our wedding day neared. Matt, true to his adventurous spirit, squeezed in a six-inch bluebird powder day with friends before the ceremony, narrowly making it to the chapel on time.

As I walked toward Matt, my heart swelled with love for the handsome, thoughtful man who had captured my soul. From the moment I first saw Matt, something inexplicable whispered that he would one day be my husband. During our courtship, he had shown nothing but unwavering integrity, genuine kindness, and a character that set him apart. I knew when he said, "I do," he meant it, no matter what lay ahead.

The evening was magical—a winter wonderland under a full moon and clear, starry sky. Guests savored New England lobster rolls and buttery Southern grits as longtime local après-ski bar singer Jonny Mogambo and his five-piece band energized the crowd with a lively mix of reggae and Grateful Dead classics.

Wrapped in a white fur stole over my strapless gown, and Matt in his traditional tuxedo, we slow-danced to Jonny's rendition of *Brokedown Palace*, as we reflected on the worlds we'd come since we first left home and our love that was too deep for words.

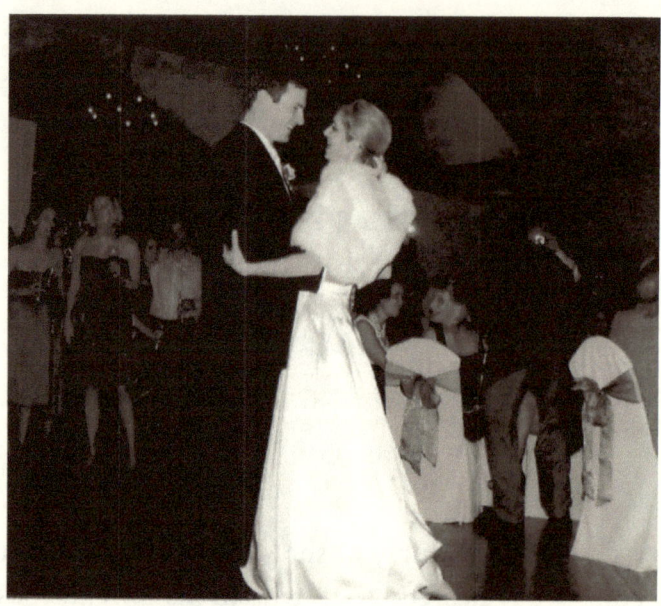

Our first dance to Brokedown Palace.

As we prepared to leave the reception, Devon, Matt's best friend, approached us with a gift in hand. Their friendship was forged as co-captains on the Middlebury baseball team, where they played pitcher and catcher—a relationship built on trust, communication, and an almost instinctive understanding of each other's tendencies. This bond, one of sport's closest, endured both on and off the field. Their connection followed them from Vermont to Colorado, where Devon now worked as a journalist for the *Summit Daily*, a regional newspaper serving the neighboring ski resorts. With his sharp eye and knack for reading people, Devon could size someone up in an instant.

Our first meeting, however, was anything but relaxed. Devon checked me out by literally sniffing the air around me before launching into what felt like an interrogation for one of his articles. I quickly realize he was vetting me, determined to ensure I was a good match for his co-captain.

Now, as we hugged him goodbye, the intensity of that first meeting was a distant memory. Handing us a white bag, Devon said warmly,

"I wanted to make sure you opened this before your trip."

Inside were two iPods, each pre-loaded with carefully curated reggae playlists. "I figured you could use some authentic vibes to set the tone," he explained with a grin. Devon had grown up on the island of St. John, and knowing Matt's sincere passion for good music, he made sure the gift reflected both their shared love for the genre.

I couldn't help but feel grateful—not just for the thoughtful gift, but for the hard-won blessing behind it. Devon's approval felt like the final seal of confidence that I was, indeed, the right partner for Matt.

A limousine carried us away to begin our new life together: first to retrieve Sadie, our beloved dog, from my parents' house and then back home. We popped champagne and reflected on the perfect day—the laughter, the vows, the promise of forever.

On Monday, we embarked on our eagerly anticipated honeymoon to the lush, twin-island nation of Saint Kitts & Nevis in the Caribbean. As we stepped off the plane, a wave of warm, humid air enveloped us. Towering palm trees swayed under a brilliant sapphire sky. The white-sand beach stretched before us, powdery and warm beneath our feet, while the waves sparkled with sunlight. The transition from the crisp, alpine air of Vail to this tropical Eden felt surreal—like walking from a snow globe into a postcard.

Eager to soak up the equatorial sun, I disregarded Matt's suggestion to wear sunscreen on the first day. However, my enthusiasm for tanning my winter-white skin soon turned to discomfort, as I resembled a lobster within hours. Determined not to let my sunburn ruin our getaway, I spent the next couple of days clad in pants and long sleeves and seeking shade, though the pain served as a cautionary reminder of my carelessness. Despite the minor setback, we reveled in the surrounding paradise. A personal highlight was holding a real diaper-wearing spider monkey—its small fingers curling around my wrist as its expressive eyes darted curiously between us. I'd always dreamed of having one as a pet, and for a few fleeting minutes, it felt like a childhood wish had come to life.

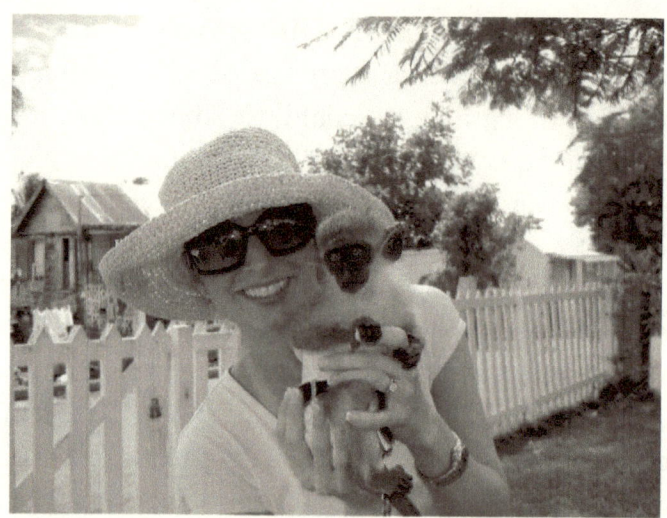

Our honeymoon in St. Kitts.

Midway through our trip, curiosity led me to switch on the television. Disconnected from current events, I was intrigued to catch up on news from the US. The headlines featured the sudden death of Anna Nicole Smith, the high-profile 39-year-old Playboy Bunny, who gained an iconic reputation after marrying an elderly oil tycoon. Speculation surrounding her passing—from dieting products to pharmaceuticals—had everyone wondering what had caused her heart to suddenly stop. I pondered how people can have such life and then cease to exist. After a few minutes, I switched off the television and returned to our honeymoon bliss. For some reason I couldn't explain, it was a story I felt connected to.

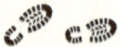

Valentine's Day 2007 began like any other, but as newlyweds, it carried extra meaning. Rather than going out to celebrate, Matt and I planned a cozy evening at home. Fresh from our wedding and exotic vacation, a low-key night felt right. I dressed in one of my favorite green sweaters that brought out the color in my eyes, paired it with brown dress pants and high-heeled leather boots, and off I went.

Before work, I stopped at the grocery store for dinner ingredients: steak, fresh vegetables, and Valentine's card featuring a dog wagging its tail, reflecting our beloved Sadie. A few chocolates and conversation hearts rounded out the gesture. I left the groceries in the car, knowing the cold temperature would keep things fresh until I could return at lunch to refrigerate them. Then, I headed to my second day at the Vail Valley Partnership, where we were launching a new client database.

The office, nestled in a familiar part of Vail, sat across from the chapel where we had exchanged our vows eleven days earlier and near the condo where I had spent countless childhood vacations. The scent of wood-smoke and thin alpine air stirred memories of those early years-so vivid they felt like yesterday.

I could still feel the thrill of skiing as a child: four years old, barreling downhill with wild hair flying beneath my green-and-white Snoopy hat and child-sized goggles. My navy floral one-piece snowsuit unzipped flapped as I raced, mittens dangling from strings in the wind. Pure, unfiltered joy coursed through me, the mountain wide open and endless beneath my skis. There was no fear, only freedom. Even at that tender age, I sensed a deep connection forming with the mountains. It was more than love; it was belonging. That bond had shaped me then, and it was guiding me still.

Standing in that same valley, my dreams were materializing. The life I'd imagined living in Vail, one of adventure and freedom, was no longer a distant hope. It was reality—as if the mountains had always called me to this moment.

The day's agenda included a training session, originally planned for a location ten miles away, had moved at the last minute to our office's conference room. It seemed like a minor detail. Sitting beside two new coworkers, we made small talk before the presentation began. I listened intently, intrigued by the possibilities of the new system.

Then, without warning, everything went dark. I collapsed in my chair, my body convulsing.

CHAPTER 3
On the Edge of Life

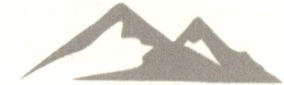

One second, I had been speaking. The next, a wave of dizziness had swallowed me into darkness. The last words spoken were about a 'streamlined solution'—an ironic phrase, considering what came next.

My coworkers' voices shifted from alarm to chaos. To the onlookers, it appeared I was having a seizure—my limbs clenching and jerking in a terrifying rhythm.

"Who knows CPR?" Mike, our executive director, shouted, his voice cutting through the confusion.

Down the hall, Sue Froeschle, a composed and adventurous longtime Girl Scout in her mid-fifties, heard the call.

"I do," she affirmed calmly, assuming it was a question about renewing her training certificate.

"We need you in the conference room NOW!" Mike barked.

Only then did Sue grasp the urgency. She took off running, heart pounding and mentally steering herself. As she reached the doorway, she asked, "Have you called 911?"

"They're on the line," Mike replied, waving her in.

As Sue entered the room, she heard my gasping—ragged, reflexive, and terrifying. The sounds weren't signs of life, but the body's last desperate attempt to breathe.

"Is it a seizure?" someone asked, watching my twitching limbs and hearing the unnatural respirations.

No one recognized the signs. It was cardiac arrest.

In the conference room, Sue immediately understood the gravity of the situation. I lay motionless—pale, lips tinted blue—clear signs of oxygen deprivation. "We need to do CPR!", she said without hesitation.

Scott, the HR director who had just processed my paperwork the day before, stepped forward. "Sue, I had training in high school. You handle compressions—I'll give the breaths."

At that moment, a team formed, not by design, but by instinct, training, and sheer determination to save my life. Together, they launched into the fight for my survival.

Coworkers dashed outside to flag down firefighters from the nearby station.

Inside, Sue knelt beside me, her face set with resolve. She laced her fingers and placed her hands on my chest to begin compressions.

"One, two, three . . ." Sue counted aloud. Each push was forceful and measured. The heels of her hands drove down with purpose, feeling my ribs shift under the pressure. Sweat beaded on her forehead, but she kept going, her voice steady.

After thirty compressions, Scott seamlessly stepped in, tilted my head and delivered two breaths. He watched for a rise in my chest, any hint of life.

The cycle continued—thirty compressions, two breaths—a relentless effort against time. The air filled with the rhythm of counting—hope battling fear.

Across the street at the Fire Station, Captain Spell and Lieutenant Sutter spotted commotion from coworkers outside. Spell was a seasoned first responder with a wife and son about my age. Sutter was young and also new to marriage. Still, instinct kicked in. They ran toward the building. Though neither knew me, something about the situation felt personal.

By my side, they seamlessly took over. Their presence brought visible relief to Sue and Scott, who had kept me alive for nearly five excruciating minutes. Now, trained emergency responders were in charge.

Paramedics arrived next. The lead, Graham—a contemporary in age with a young wife—exuded calm authority. "Continue CPR, expose the chest, and prepare for defibrillation," he instructed.

In practiced coordination, they cut away my clothing and placed the defibrillator pads on my bare chest. The monitor displayed ventricular fibrillation—V-fib—a chaotic, deadly rhythm.

Graham quickly assessed the situation and made a deliberate decision. Based on my presentation, he departed from the standard protocol, shocking me at 200 joules instead of the usual 160. "Clear!" he called. My body jolted with the force of the first shock, but my heart did not convert. The erratic rhythm persisted.

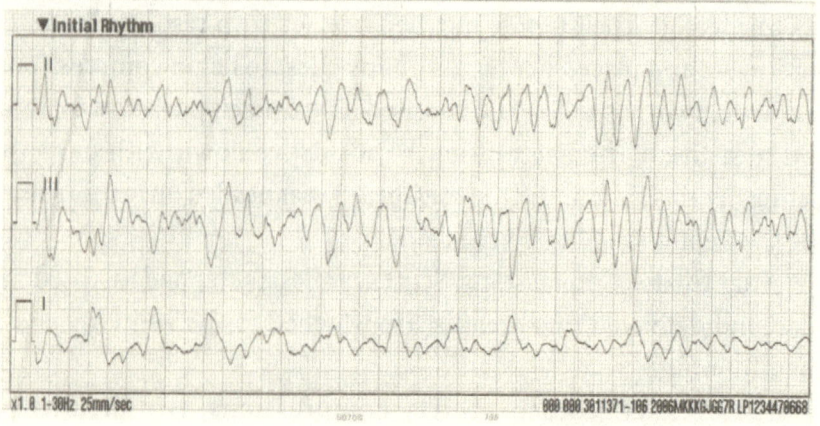

Ventricular fibrillation, EKG reading from February 14, 2007.

CPR resumed immediately. The team moved swiftly by starting an IV and pushing amiodarone to help stabilize my heart's electrical activity.

Two minutes later, Graham delivered a second shock. This time, the response was different. A strong pulse returned that was fragile, but unmistakably there. I was alive.

With no time to spare, they began the next phase: transport. The stairway to exit the building was narrow, so they used a backboard to navigate the tight angles, a firefighter on each corner. Graham crouched below to support the team, hauling the full load of medical gear. They moved me up the stairs, through the falling snow and into a waiting ambulance for a short drive to our small-town hospital, Vail Health.

The fight wasn't over, but for a moment, there was hope.

Upon our arrival, the situation took a sharp turn for the worse. My heart stopped again.

CHAPTER 4
In Sickness and in Health

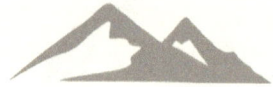

Matt must have felt a swirl of emotions that Valentine's Day—overwhelmed, yet strangely content. We'd just rebound from our honeymoon days earlier. While the time spent in Saint Kitts had been blissful, it also meant a backlog of work awaited him upon his return. But he didn't mind. Matt was a hard worker and determined to support our shared dreams.

As an up-and-coming realtor, Matt juggled twenty to thirty real estate listings. His day blurred in a flurry of phone calls and deal-making at the office. However, he noticed a missed call from me on his phone. Dialing my number, he was taken aback when a voice other than mine answered the phone.

"This is Allison from Lynn's work. Lynn passed out," came the unexpected news.

Concern etched into his voice, Matt responded, "Low blood sugar maybe, or dehydration?"

"We called 911, and the ambulance is on its way," Allison replied.

Her words moved him to action, Matt hurried to his car, only to discover his recently upgraded Jeep Grand Cherokee refusing to start. Luckily, Matt was just patient enough, and with one more try, the engine came roaring to life. Rushing to my workplace, he arrived to find the ambulance had already departed, leaving bystanders behind a tense cloud of worry.

"They just took her away, but she was breathing," Allison informed him, handing over my purse and brown high-heeled leather boots.

With barely any information, there was a growing sense of urgency. Matt jumped back in his car and headed straight to the emergency room, his mind racing with concern.

Next, Allison got hold of my dad. "Hi, is this Lynn's dad?" came her hesitant voice.

"Yes," he replied, a tremor of concern coloring his tone.

Allison's words pierced through his calm: "I'm so sorry to tell you, but something just happened to Lynn. The paramedics are working on her and taking her to Vail Health."

In a rush, my dad tracked down my mom at work and delivered the news that would change their lives. "It's Lynn. We need to go now. She's headed to the hospital. Maybe a seizure?"

My mom shot up, barely nodding to her coworker as she raced out the door.

Prayers tumbled from her lips between breaths as they rushed to the car. On the way, my mom made frantic calls to ask everyone she could think of to pray for me, her newlywed daughter. A memory flashed in her mind—the uncertain days after my birth. She knew this wasn't just a seizure; it was her worst fear coming to life.

Matt and my parents arrived at Vail Health simultaneously. Motion blurred the scene—nurses in scrubs darting past, phones ringing, monitors beeping. The fluorescent lights buzzed faintly above them, casting a cold, clinical glow across the room.

Dr. Podgorny, the emergency physician on duty, shocked and restarted my heart again. He and Graham worked together to intubate me, stabilize my vitals, and run imaging and tests to assess the damage.

While the medical team fought to keep my heart beating, my family stood frozen in the sterile corridor, separated by a wall of doctors. Unbeknownst to them, my heart had stopped again. Behind closed doors, the team was working urgently to prepare me for transport to a hospital in Denver that could provide the specialized cardiac care I desperately needed.

Matt couldn't sit. He paced the tiled floor, his boots squeaking faintly with each turn. The graveness of his vows—to love, to cherish, in sickness and in health—pressed down on him, heavier with every minute that passed. His palms were damp. He rubbed them against his jeans, then ran a hand through his hair, eyes flicking toward every door that opened, hoping for answers, fearing the worst.

Dr. Podgorny stepped away to update my family.

"Is she going to make it?" Matt's voice cracked, desperation bleeding through. "Please—just tell me she's going to be okay."

Dr. Podgorny exhaled slowly, eyes steady but solemn. "She's alive," he said, letting the words settle. "She suffered sudden cardiac arrest. We got her heart beating again, but . . . her status is uncertain."

The bombshell was immediate. As the news dawned on him, my dad's interjection cut through the silence. "Heart issues." His words pointed to the hidden cloud that hovered over my past. This revelation shook Matt to the core, casting a shadow of doubt over everything he thought about his wife's well-being—young, thin, physically capable.

Twenty-seven and seemingly healthy, I defied the usual image of a cardiac patient, puzzling even the staff. My mother, who had stepped away to pray for a miracle, then returned to answer questions about my medical history. When Matt was asked repeatedly about illicit drugs, he answered firmly, "No, no drugs," holding his patience as best he could.

In the emergency room, the air smelled faintly of alcohol wipes and bleach, as machines hummed in the background with a steady, mechanical rhythm. A male nurse stood at my bedside. He turned to my mom and asked softly, "Do you know how to braid hair?"

His voice was calm, almost reverent, a gentle counterpoint to the tension in the room.

"She has such beautiful hair," he added, brushing a strand away from my face with practiced care, as if honoring something sacred in the ordinary.

With trembling hands, my mom braided my hair, her touch tender against my cool skin.

The nurse continued, "You should go home and get a change of clothes," he said. "Grab whatever you need. This will not be a short stay."

The words hung in the air like a warning bell. Until then, they'd been operating on adrenaline—barely breathing, barely comprehending. But now, reality was setting in. I wasn't going home tonight. Maybe not for a long time, if ever.

A higher level of care was required—and fast. However, the blizzard outside grounded the Flight for Life helicopter that had been called to quicken the transport to a larger hospital with cardiac specialists.

An alternate decision was made. I needed to be driven to Denver. The team carefully loaded me into the ambulance, ready for the precarious transport. This trip, under normal conditions, is two to three hours, but in a winter storm, it could be many hours more if one or both of the mountain passes between Vail and Denver closed, leaving the crew on their own and me in their hands.

With no time to lose, paramedics Graham, Dawn, and Jenn began their high-stakes journey, determined to reach the advanced care I needed with urgency and resolve.

As my family watched the crew pull away, the events of the day sent my mother back in time.

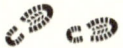

1979—Fort Worth, Texas

My birth completed my parents' vision of a perfect family. For a few days, I was a quiet baby, sleeping soundly through the night. But just six days after birth, everything changed—the first glimpse of a heart condition that wouldn't fully reveal itself until decades later.

My mom's parents, Gammy and Papa T, were staying with us to

help with my sister, Margaret, while my mom cared for me. Gammy, ever-observant, noticed a faint blue tinge on my fingers. She frowned, concerned. "They're not the right color. Olga, come look!"

Initially, my mom brushed off Gammy's worry, but her insistence led them to the emergency room at Cook Children's Hospital in Fort Worth, Texas. Late in the evening, my mom and Gammy entered the quaint, Italian-style medical facility. They were ushered into a partitioned room where a small defibrillator with infant pads hung above the examination table. My mom watched as the doctor checked me over with cold, unfamiliar hands.

After inspecting me, the doctor suggested my mom dilute her breast milk, thinking it was "too rich." Though skeptical, she had no way to fact-check and reluctantly followed his advice.

Back home, she hoped the instructions would help, but Gammy's watchful eye remained on the entire situation. The faint blueness lingered, nagging at my mom. Filled with doubt, she finally turned to our family pediatrician, Dr. Nyman. His familiar, child-friendly office felt like a haven, and as she shared her concerns, she hoped he'd have the answers the emergency doctor didn't.

As Dr. Nyman listened through his stethoscope, a shadow crossed his face. With calm urgency, he said, "I want you to see a friend of mine . . . *now!*"

Confused, my mom asked why. His response was dark: "Lynn's heart is beating so fast that I can't count it."

The seriousness hit hard. She called my dad, preparing him to meet us at Dr. Tierney's office—a leading pediatric cardiologist at Cook Children's Hospital, a rare specialty in those days. My mom then raced through Friday evening traffic, arriving just in time. We were Dr. Tierney's last appointment, and he quickly realized that no one would leave soon.

The hospital buzzed as nurses and doctors worked swiftly. My mom, still weak from delivery, felt disoriented by the unfolding crisis and antiseptic smells. My dad paced restlessly, tapping and fidgeting, while my mom took in every detail of the waiting room—nervously watching the door, longing to hold me and reassure me that everything would be all right; but, I lay exposed under bright hospital lights, surrounded by foreign faces and sounds.

When Dr. Tierney finally came out, his grave expression said it all. "The initial treatments to slow her heartbeat failed, and a different approach is necessary. The proposed procedure involves shocking her heart to restore normal rhythm," he explained.

The memory of the small defibrillator paddles my mother had seen on her first visit to the hospital concerning my discolored fingers flashed in her mind.

"Mrs. Griffin?" he continued, "We need your permission to proceed, but you should know it carries the risk of . . . death," Dr. Tierney said, gently handing her the papers she would need to sign.

The word "death" struck her; the acuteness of the decision sinking in as she hesitated. Still haunted by the device on the wall, she picked up the pen and, with a trembling hand, signed: Olga Griffin.

The electrical shock made burn marks on my delicate infant chest, and, unfortunately, the defibrillation proved ineffective. My resilient heart continued to throb, like a hummingbird trapped in a jar. The unfolding ordeal was devastating my parents' hopes and dreams.

CHAPTER 5
Miracles in the Storm

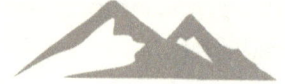

The ambulance plowed carefully through falling snow en route to Presbyterian St. Luke's Hospital (PSL). On duty that night was Dr. Fred Miller, a renowned electrophysiologist and one of the top specialists in Colorado known for being on call during high-profile visits—most recently Vice President Dick Cheney. Dr. Miller and his team were ready and waiting for our arrival.

Jenn focused on the road ahead, navigating treacherous conditions: low visibility, high winds, and worsening snow. Weather advisories urged all drivers to stay off the roads, warning that conditions would only deteriorate. But this was life or death.

In the back of the ambulance, Graham remained steady, his attention locked on my care. He wasn't alone. Dawn was there to assist with the more complex aspects of the transfer, managing ventilators, IV pumps, and critical care equipment. Together, they worked in tandem, to ensure my survival.

Dr. Miller and the trauma team met us at the doors when we reached PSL. Graham seamlessly transitioned care, recounting every detail of my condition and their interventions along the way. I was now in the hands of one of the best cardiac specialists in the state, entering the next phase of survival.

The fluorescent hospital lights revealed my battered body. I was placed in an induced coma, unaware of the intense situation that had unfolded and the storm still ahead. A new life had begun, altering my existence in ways no one could yet imagine.

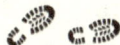

With each passing mile, the uncertainty of the crisis bore down on my mom and dad. My father's hands clenched the steering wheel, while my mother was on the phone with medical staff, trying to answer urgent questions. The quest to determine why my heart stopped on this day, Valentine's Day 2007, continued.

"We need to know about her honeymoon," they pressed, hoping for clues that might explain my sudden collapse.

Scrambling for answers, she fumbled through half-told stories, confusion clouding her thoughts. The snowfall thickened, visibility shrank, and silence filled the car. Her mind drifted to Matt, likely lost in his own blizzard of disbelief and helplessness. The normalcy of our lives had been shattered in an instant.

Meanwhile, Matt raced home to gather essentials and our dog, Sadie. With her resting calmly in his lap, he pressed through the increasing snow toward Denver, replaying every moment in his head, searching for clues he didn't have.

The Eisenhower Tunnel offered a brief shelter in the storm, a two-mile stretch of snow-free pavement. He made it through just before the road closed behind him.

Finally, at PSL, Matt and my parents were reunited. Friends gathered too, offering a presence in the face of so many unknowns.

In a corridor just outside the emergency room, they waited. Inside, doctors worked with urgent precision.

About an hour later, two physicians came to provide a status report. One of them spoke sharply: "In addition to cardiac arrest, she has a severe blood clot in her leg."

The words hit hard.

"We're going to try medication to break it up. But if that doesn't work, we'll need to amputate. As her husband, I need your signature."

Matt didn't hesitate.

"Yes. Clear it. Take her leg. Do whatever it takes to save her."

Another doctor stepped in. "It's extremely rare to see this in someone so young. Is there anything?"

"I know," Matt interrupted. "None of this makes sense."

The medications weren't working. The clot remained. Amputation looked like the only option. Matt's heart clenched under the magnitude of the decision, but he never wavered.

This is 'til death do us part,' he told himself. And if I lived without a leg, so be it. He just wanted me to survive. "Would you like to see her before we take her into surgery?"

He nodded.

At my bedside, Matt and my parents stood in stunned silence. My body was pale, motionless beneath the sheets. My mom slowly lifted the white covering. Her heart dropped. My dad couldn't bear the sight and left the room.

My leg was grotesquely swollen—the size of an elephant's—purple, cold, and unrecognizable.

At that moment, she turned to Matt.

"Put your hand on her leg," she whispered.

They bowed their heads. "Lord, save this leg." Their prayer wasn't polished—it was raw and real. A last plea for help.

As they returned to the waiting room, my mom's eyes landed on a *Reader's Digest* Christmas issue. The title jumped off the page: "Real-Life Miracles."

"Matt," she said, her voice hushed, "I think this is for us."

Doctors and nurses drifted in and out, delivering updates no one could fully make sense of.

The previously brash, barrel-chested doctor with a bulldog demeanor, approached my mom.

"Mrs. Griffin, your daughter likely won't make it."

His tone was flat, his eyes unflinching. "If she survives, she'll have brain damage. They are preparing to remove her leg now."

My mom looked him straight in the eye.

"Do you know how many people are praying for her right now?"

Not expecting such a confident response, he blinked. Silently, he turned and walked away.

1979—Fort Worth, Texas

Later that night, shortly after my birth, Gammy and Papa T drove my mom home. My dad stayed behind, unwilling to leave my side.

Back at the house, everything felt surreal. The silence was unnerving. My mom collapsed into bed as if trying to wake from a nightmare, hoping to find her healthy daughter safe in the next room.

But that wasn't her reality. My mom realized then that she could not save me. Her strength had vanished. She felt powerless.

So, she surrendered.

"Lord," she cried out into the dark, "save my daughter's life!"

In that sacred space between fear and faith, promises spilled from her heart.

"No matter what happens tonight," she whispered, "I trust you. If you take her, I know she will be with you. But if You let her live, may her life be Yours."

A peace enveloped her. It wasn't a promise of outcome, just enough calm to let her rest.

She drifted off, only to be jolted awake by the piercing ring of the phone on the wall. Frozen in the hallway, afraid to answer, she listened as Papa T picked it up.

"Hello?" he whispered, voice rough from fatigue.

A long pause followed.

"I see," he murmured.

My mom burst into the room, hair undone and eyes wide, bracing for tragedy or mercy.

"Lynn is going to be alright," Papa T said. "They got her heart rate down. Dr. Tierney said it took three injections in her forehead. The third one finally worked."

Tears spilled freely. Relief crashed over her. A Bible verse stirred in her soul: "For I know the plans I have for you," declares the Lord, "plans to prosper you and not to harm you, plans to give you hope and a future" (Jeremiah 29:11).

The following day, as they prepared to return to the hospital, Papa T handed Gammy a Polaroid camera. No words were exchanged. Years ago, they'd lost their first child shortly after birth. Only Papa T had held the baby. No photo, no keepsake had ever existed. This time, he wanted something tangible—just in case.

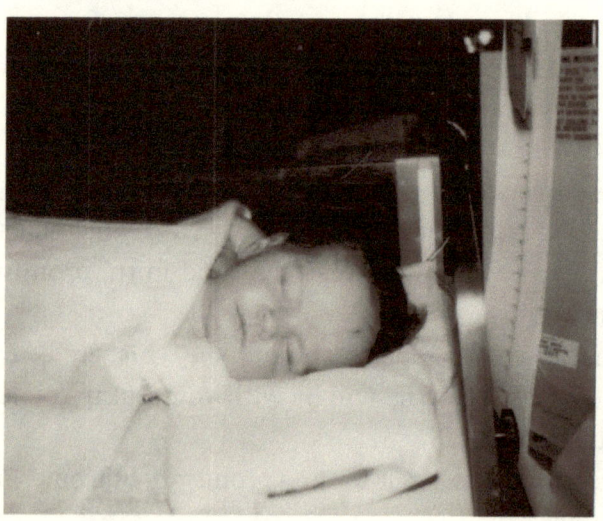

In the incubator at the NICU.

The Neonatal Intensive Care Unit (NICU) was unfamiliar territory, sterile, still, and heavy with uncertainty. Behind clear incubators lay tiny, fragile lives tethered to machines. My mom and Gammy ambled past rows of infants, each one fighting their own battles.

Many were barely two or three pounds, bodies swallowed by tubes. It was a world most people never saw, where grief and hope lived side by side.

At seven pounds, six ounces, and twenty-one inches, I was the largest baby there. A section of my forehead had been shaved for the injections, but I lay peacefully, eyes closed, recovering from the trauma of the night before.

A nurse approached. "Would you like to hold her?"

"Oh yes, thank you," my mom whispered.

As she cradled me, questions filled her mind. *Will she be able to run and play? Could this happen again? How do we raise a child with a heart that could break at any moment?*

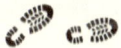

Now in Denver, as my family waited in tense silence, a doctor entered the room, this time with astonishment on his face.

"Mr. and Mrs. Griffin, Mr. Blake," he began. "Lynn's leg has . . . completely turned around. The clot has cleared."

Stunned silence.

"No amputation?" my mom asked, barely breathing.

"Not at this time. We're still watching closely. She's in critical condition. We don't know what recovery will look like or what kind of brain damage may be present. But for now, you can rest."

Rest. It was a word they hadn't considered in hours.

As they prepared to leave the hospital that night, my mom ran into Dr. Miller in the hallway.

"You're Lynn's mom, right?" he asked.

She nodded.

"I just want you to know," he said, "we never imagined her leg would turn around like that."

Outside, the night was quiet. Stars glittered across the cold sky.

And in that silence, my mother knew. A miracle was performed.

CHAPTER 6
Uncertain Future

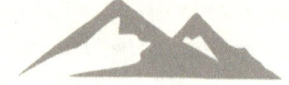

1979—Fort Worth, Texas

The incubator became my crib with its transparent plastic walls and harsh fluorescent lights defining the edges of my newborn world. My parents' routines disappeared, replaced by hours spent in the NICU, keeping vigil, desperate for clarity.

Dr. Tierney diagnosed me with ventricular tachycardia—V-tach—a dangerous arrhythmia where the heart's lower chambers beat so fast, they can't pump blood efficiently. He explained brief episodes might be harmless, but prolonged rhythms like mine starve the body of oxygen and can be fatal.

He shared my records with specialists nationwide, yet no one could explain the cause. The unknown diagnosis left my family unbalanced, clinging to hope while bracing for the worst.

After a harrowing week, my heart finally settled into a steady rhythm. The doctors, satisfied with my progress, released me to go home. Relief came with additional responsibilities. My parents' lives now revolved around my medications. Though bone-tired, my mom still woke at odd hours to dose me, too afraid of what might happen if she missed one.

At home, we slipped into a fragile routine. Doctor visits became regular events, yet my mom still had a sense that this wasn't over. That feeling stayed with her, quiet and persistent.

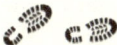

Two days after my cardiac arrest, I still lay in an induced coma. My family, unsure if I would ever wake up, began preparing themselves for what life would look like without me in it.

News of my condition spread quickly. Waves of support followed.

Bouquets started arriving, coloring the hospital room with bursts of hopefulness amid the quiet dread. Each arrangement said what words could not.

Relatives traveled in to stand watch. My sister Margaret came with her husband, Billy, and their two-year-old son, Will. My in-laws, Joanne and David, arrived, along with Uncle Jeff and Aunt Barbara. Their presence was heavy, their suitcases packed with funeral clothes. Jeff, a doctor, knew more than most how bad the odds were—less than ten percent survive. The joy of our wedding, still fresh in memory, already felt like a distant dream.

Billy did his best to lighten the room. Armed with Valentine's Day clearance decorations, he hung heart-shaped garlands, tissue chandeliers, and three magnetic monkeys on my bed. The irony wasn't lost on my family—Valentine hearts hung around a room with people fighting to keep mine alive.

Little Will brightened the mood. He tugged on cords and explored buttons, giggling, blissfully unaware of the quiet panic surrounding him. His innocence was a gift for my family. People took turns offering comfort and making sure Matt stayed grounded. He was holding it together, but only on the outside.

Devon, who had been the last to say goodbye at our wedding, now handed Matt a letter, his words genuine and honest. What had been a joyous send-off now felt like a reunion no one had wanted.

Adrienne, my best friend since high school, couldn't make it back so soon after the wedding. Instead, she sent her grandparents—who were like family—and our childhood friend from Denver in her place, bearing flowers and a batch of warm chocolate chip cookies.

The most meaningful gift of all: a purple polka-dot robe sent from my sister-in-law. Draped over my hospital gown, it offered dignity and warmth, a little piece of composure in the lack of privacy.

The room was quickly transformed. Cards, stuffed animals, and flowers filled every surface. The sterile space became a garden of love and hope for survival.

But my body told a different story.

Deep bruises marred my pale skin. My eyes remained shut, unmoved by voices or touch. I lay motionless—suspended in the unknown.

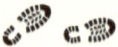

On the third day, a slight improvement: the doctors began easing me out of the coma. Survivors of cardiac arrest often face cognitive damage, and my prognosis loomed. As sedation lifted, I grew extremely agitated from the tube in my throat, which prevented me from speaking and breathing on my own.

The first hurdle was removing the breathing tube. As I stirred, unable to speak, panic set in. My hands clawed at the tube lodged in my throat.

The removal was excruciating. My throat spasmed and burned, leaving me coughing and gagging. But I was breathing. I was alive.

The medical team stayed close, waiting until I was stable.

My eyes half-lidded. Speech was raw. Aches radiated from my chest. My body was heavy. Each movement took effort. Though I couldn't understand it, the trauma was apparent and discombobulating.

Questions surfaced in my foggy mind. Why was I here? What had happened?

I couldn't remember any of it.

Despite my relatively stable condition and promise of cognitive function, the next phase of treatment transpired.

The doctors recommended a device, an implantable cardioverter defibrillator, or ICD. Its job was to maintain a normal heart rhythm and to monitor and intervene if it detected a life-threatening arrhythmia like V-fib. If that happened, the ICD would first try to pace my heart back into rhythm. If pacing failed, it would deliver a powerful shock to restore normal electrical function.

If V-fib were sustained, I'd likely lose consciousness before the shock hit and wouldn't feel a thing. The device should step in like an invisible paramedic, who would deliver the jolt I needed before anyone even recognized what happened.

However, if the device misfired, shocking me while I was fully awake, that was a different story. I'd feel it. It's not the most excruciating pain, but it's sharp, sudden, and unforgettable. Like getting kicked in the chest from the inside out, leaving you breathless, stunned, and instantly on edge, wondering why it happened.

The good news is you don't see it coming. There's no countdown, no moment to brace yourself, no expecting it like you would a scheduled treatment.

Getting shocked by the ICD was one of those things doctors encouraged me not to think about too much. But that was impossible, because the scenario was possible.

Regardless, the ICD was a safeguard, a medical necessity to resume anything resembling a normal life. But the thought of living with it? That terrified me.

I begged not to have the procedure.

The idea of having a zapping battery inside my body, one that fires off jolts without warning, made me feel vulnerable and uneasy. What if it malfunctioned? What if it shocked me when I didn't need it—or didn't work when I did? The thought of the device protruding beneath my skin unsettled me. I worried about how it would affect my appearance, my identity, even my daily life. Would I still be able to travel, exercise, go through security, ski?

While it offered protection, it also represented a loss of control—and a permanent reminder that my heart had failed me once before.

My fear was louder than reason. The decision had already been made.

Dr. Miller led the operation.

Once sedated, surgeons threaded wires through my veins to connect the device to my heart. The muscle was cut to tuck the ICD just beneath my left clavicle. Once everything was in place, V-fib was intentionally triggered to ensure the ICD responded appropriately.

When it was done, a small scar marked the spot, commemorating what I'd survived—and now required.

The recovery was painful. Every breath tugged at my chest. I couldn't lift my arm. Even lying down was uncomfortable.

But beneath the discomfort was something deeper: an awareness that my body now relied on something outside of itself to survive.

The ICD wasn't just metal and wires.

It was my lifeline.

Each heartbeat echoed the words I couldn't ignore: I need a miracle every day just to stay alive.

CHAPTER 7
Cognitive Fog

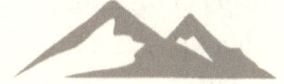

1982—Fort Worth, Texas

After three years of positive reports and no signs of tachycardia, Dr. Tierney recommended advanced testing in Houston. The timing wasn't ideal—Easter was approaching, and we had plans to visit Gammy and Papa T in Mississippi. But urgency took precedence. My mom and I packed up, determined to fit everything into the tight schedule.

I was scheduled for a procedure under the care of Dr. Gordon, a young cardiologist with an eccentric air, bowtie and all. Though unconventional, he had a strong reputation. My mom felt reassured knowing esteemed colleagues trusted him.

"We'll be performing a heart catheterization," he explained. "A thin tube will be inserted into a blood vessel in her groin and threaded into her heart. We'll measure pressures, check for damage, and assess blood flow." Then he added, almost too casually, "To complete the test, we'll need to stop and restart her heart."

My mom's face stiffened. Her eye twitched involuntarily. In the early '80s, this was far from routine, especially for a toddler.

Sensing her fear, Dr. Gordon added gently, "She's in the best hands. We'll take care of her."

She nodded and signed the forms, her hand trembling. Once again, she was signing off on risks she couldn't even name.

Sedated and wheeled away, I disappeared down the hall. My mom was led to the waiting room—her least favorite place in any hospital. The vinyl chairs, the sterile lighting, the silence—all of it suffocating.

She found a seat and buried her head in her hands.

"God, please ... just keep her breathing." Her words were not elegant, but desperate. A mother's plea from the deepest part of her soul.

"I give her to You. You love her even more than I do."

She was surrendering—offering what she couldn't hold, trusting what she couldn't see.

Each time the door opened, every head in the waiting room turned.

When Dr. Gordon finally entered, he approached with a smile. "It went well," he said. "We found only a small area of concern in a remote part of her heart. There's barely any damage at all."

Relief washed over my mom.

"So, she'll be able to live a normal life?" she asked.

"Yes," he replied. "Everything should be fine."

That night was long. Keeping a restless three-year-old off a leg where a catheter had been inserted wasn't easy. By morning, we were ready to go, armed with good news and renewed optimism.

When we arrived at Gammy and Papa T's in Mississippi, the Easter celebration was especially joyful. As I darted across the lawn in search of eggs, my mom let herself believe that maybe, just maybe, the storm was finally behind us.

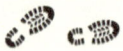

Decades later, that medical charge returned, this time with more critical symptoms and side effects.

Pete and Whitney, close friends who were keeping Sadie and visited often, became unwitting participants in my short-term memory lapses. Before the wedding, old photos were gathered, including one of Pete and Matt in their early ski bum days in Vail. I couldn't believe how youthfully thin Pete looked and eagerly shared the discovery during a visit.

The next time they stopped by, I brought it up again, forgetting I'd already told him. "There's this photo of you…" I started.

Pete smiled. "Let me guess, you found one where I'm skinny?"

I laughed it off, but inside, I felt the sting. My mind looped like a scratched record, replaying thoughts as if for the first time.

At first, I chalked it up to stress and exhaustion. Everyone forgets things, right? But the scenario played out for a third time! The humor faded into quiet dread. Had I suffered more brain damage than we realized.

Matt was steady. "You've been through a lot," he reminded me gently. "Give yourself a break."

Forgetting a conversation was one thing. Struggling to recall parts of a life-altering trauma was something else entirely.

The days after my collapse were a blur, like trying to watch life through frosted glass. Entire conversations vanished as if they'd never happened. I'd begin a sentence with purpose, only to lose the thread halfway through. I couldn't hold on to thoughts long enough to feel grounded.

Inside, I was panicking. How long would this last? Would it get worse?

People would recount things I should know, and I'd nod blankly, pretending to remember. The mental fog wasn't just frustrating—it was terrifying. It chipped away at my confidence and ability to trust my mind.

Without memories to anchor me, I felt like a visitor in my own life.

But in those moments of disorientation, the steady presence of family and friends tethered me. Their patience reminded me that even if memory faltered, love remained.

My mind was mush, but my spirit held. Each day brought a new challenge—and a new chance to move forward. The scars on my body spoke of pain, yes, but also of survival. I was still here.

What I didn't expect was how much I'd miss Sadie.

Her absence at the hospital left a hollow space I couldn't explain. Throughout my life, animals had been more than companions; they were my best friends and teachers. I connected with them in ways I struggled to connect with people. Their silent presence, free of judgment, brought unconditional acceptance.

I'd loved many furry creatures growing up, from wild raccoons to tiny hamsters. But I'd always dreamed of one companion to walk beside me through life's highs and lows. When I first saw a Cavalier King Charles Spaniel with soulful eyes and floppy ears, I knew. That was my breed.

During a season of milestones with Matt, our conversations naturally shifted to the future. One night over dinner, I mentioned wanting a dog. A Cavalier, tri-color, specifically.

That Christmas, Matt handed me a small, thin wrapped package. Inside was a book on caring for Cavaliers, along with photos of an upcoming litter.

"We get first pick," he said, smiling. "She'll be ready after our ski trip to Verbier."

My heart swelled. This wasn't just a puppy—it was a promise. A step forward. I quietly hoped it might be followed by another promise, a ring.

Six weeks later, she came home. We named her Sadie Mae.

She was tiny, delicate, and perfect. With her short snout and perfectly dotted coat, she looked like something out of a painting. Sadie went to work and ran errands with me, her tiny head poking out of a colorful designer pet bag. Raising Sadie together deepened our bond. She was more than a pet. She was our baby, a projection of what we were building: a life rooted in family and shared purpose.

While I was hospitalized, Pete and Whitney—knowing how much Sadie meant to me—hatched a plan. Despite the hospital's strict no-pet policy, they smuggled her in, a fluffy outlaw tucked into a duffel bag. Everyone was in on the plan. There were no metal detectors, no bag checks, just a quick nod to security and a casual stroll past the nurses' station. No one suspected a thing. The bag wiggled once, maybe twice, but they kept moving until they slipped quietly into my room.

The bag was unzipped. And there she was—Sadie, tail thumping, eyes wide with joy. For the first time in days, I smiled because I meant it.

Then she paused, scanning the room. Her gaze landed on me. Slowly, she stepped onto the bed and gently nestled close.

As I stroked her fur, I felt a stillness I hadn't known in days. She didn't speak, didn't need to. Her presence said it all.

For a moment, the noise, the fear, the pain, and the uncertainty faded.

Sadie comforted me.

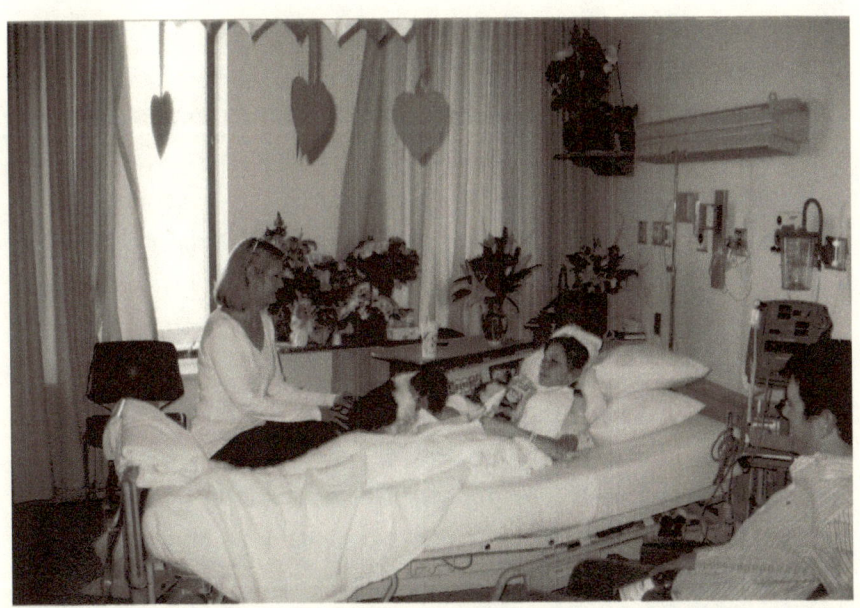

Sadie visits the hospital.

CHAPTER 8
When Heaven Is Quiet

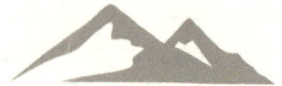

During one of the long hospital days, my mom's pastor friend stopped by with a suggestion: *90 Minutes in Heaven* by Don Piper. It told the story of a man who survived a horrific car crash and described a vivid, near-death experience, including a glimpse of heaven and his long recovery.

My dad picked up a copy, and visitors took turns reading it aloud at my bedside. The book opened with Piper's account of a head-on collision involving a semi-truck on a Texas bridge. First responders declared him dead. For the next hour and a half, he claimed to be in heaven, a place of blinding light, peace, and reunion with loved ones.

As my mom read the descriptions of heaven's beauty, something in me twisted.

"Mom, stop reading," I blurted, my voice tight and unfamiliar.

She froze. "Sure, what's wrong?"

I couldn't articulate a response. During my brush with death, I'd seen nothing. No light. No warmth. No heavenly embrace.

It unsettled me to think about the afterlife. Many talk about traveling through a tunnel, seeing a light or people that died before them, or hearing a voice say, 'It's not your time.' But I experienced nothing. That absence left a quiet dread. Was I not going to heaven? I had never truly acknowledged God, not in the way my mom had.

That doubt took me back to a night I hadn't thought about in years, November 9, 1989, the day the Berlin Wall fell. My family joined the world as everyone watched a symbol of division crumble, footage of streets under surveillance, where border guards stood motionless with weapons at the ready; the Wall was layered with spray-painted pleas, people protesting, and cries for rebellion. I saw crowds chanting in a language I couldn't understand, their voices rising in unison. It may have been a celebration culminating, but that's not what struck me. What I saw was the grief of separation and the agony of division. It lingered in their faces and shouts. And it didn't sit well with my soul.

I lay in bed, overwhelmed by fear. Questions about division, death, eternity, and God swirled in my ten-year-old mind.

I couldn't sleep. I went to my mom, seeking comfort. She opened the Bible and explained the human condition: no one is perfect, everyone falls short, and, therefore, we all will endure death at some point. Then she told me that if I asked Jesus into my heart, I could live forever in heaven. So, we prayed together in the night's quiet. Next, she handed me a pen and encouraged me to write it down as confirmation. There, in the front of my *Precious Moments* Bible, I inscribed "I asked Jesus into my HEART on November 9, 1989."

Weeks later, as Christmas approached, my mom gathered us to share some tough truths. She was worn out by the constant requests for more toys and things. "Girls, come sit down. I have something important to tell you," she said. My heart raced—I thought maybe she was going to tell us we were getting a new sibling. Instead, she looked at us gently and broke the news, "Santa Claus is not real." The holiday, she explained, had become too focused on the cultural pressure of gift-giving.

Then came our questions about the Tooth Fairy. And the Easter Bunny.

I was stunned. Thinking of any other fantastical beings, I asked her, "What about God and Jesus? Are they real?"

"Yes," she said without hesitation. "Jesus is real."

But the cracks had already formed. My belief in the unseen had been shaken. And now, lying in a hospital bed as a grown woman, those questions returned. They were no longer questions about fairy tales—they were questions about life and death.

"Lynn." My mom's voice snapped me back to the room.

"Look at me," her tone firm but loving. "This happened for a reason. God is going to use it for good. Every single thing that lined up to keep you alive wasn't random. You are a miracle."

She began listing what she saw as divine orchestration: the timing of the job, the proximity to first responders, that it happened on Valentine's Day. Then she added, almost offhandedly, "And did you know one of the firefighters who saved you was Ryan Sutter? The guy from *The Bachelorette*?"

The absurdity of it cracked something open in me. Ryan Sutter? A reality TV star helped save my life?

I laughed briefly. But then shame crept in. The thought of strangers, celebrity or not, seeing me shirtless and vulnerable felt unbearable. I yanked at the oxygen tubing, frustrated by the reminder of how fragile I'd become.

My mom believed in miracles. But I was stuck in the fear of what might happen next, what would happen when my heart stopped for good.

All I wanted was to go home and forget this ever happened.

My loved ones did everything they could to lift my spirits.

My favorite Cotton Candy, Pina Colada and Coconut Jelly Belly beans brought a burst of joy until I overdid it. My blood sugar spiked, alarming the medical staff. One nurse was prepared to administer insulin.

"She's not diabetic," Matt insisted.

The next morning, a different nurse arrived, still convinced I needed treatment. My mom stood firm. "It's the candy," she said calmly. "Just the candy."

Apparently, sugary sweets can cause glucose levels to rise so high that insulin is required to control it—who knew? I survive a cardiac arrest, and then nearly die again from a jelly bean overdose. It would've been funny if it weren't so serious.

It was a small but telling moment. Every detail of my care mattered. We had to question everything. We had to advocate—even against snack-related false alarms.

In the quiet moments between sleep, visits, meals, vitals, and blood draws, my thoughts spiraled. What if no one had been there when my heart failed? Matt would've found me lifeless. What if it had happened on the plane? Or during our remote honeymoon?

But it didn't.

It happened across the street from the Vail Fire Department. During a training session. With CPR-certified coworkers present. With Sue in the building. At exactly the right moment. And to top it off, it occurred on the heartiest heart day of the year.

I couldn't ignore the precision of it all, even if I didn't understand it.

By day six, I took my first steps. Each move was shaky—but defiant.

The doctors speculated about what had caused the arrest. A blood clot. Wedding stress. Birth control. Past arrhythmias. Or something else entirely. I thought about two other factors: an Adderall prescription and a past eating disorder. But I didn't share those details. Not yet. I wasn't ready.

"Hopefully, you'll live a normal life," they said. But even their optimism had limits. One doctor told me the hard truth: the average lifespan post cardiac arrest was seven to eight years.

The prognosis was a statistical midpoint. Most patients have severe underlying cardiac conditions, sustain significant neurological damage, and remain at high risk for future events. But data is not destiny—many live far beyond the average.

He concluded with a sliver of hope. "You're young. You might live a much longer life."

Might. That word lingered—a hope for better than average.

We'd been married less than two weeks and should still be floating in the glow of vows and dreams. Like our parents, we imagined growing old together—forty years or more of a shared life. But now, with a device stitched beneath my skin and questions lingering in every heartbeat, I couldn't help but wonder: Is the most we can hope for seven years? Can we even have children?

The next few days in the hospital dragged on, each one blurring into the next. I felt restless, convinced I was well enough to go home. But time moved slowly, measured not by clocks, but by routine checks, the beeping of monitors, and the shuffle of nurses.

Frustration with the confinement was wearing on me. My wedding manicure, once pristine, had turned into a reminder of how much had changed. The acrylic was lifting, the polish chipped, and I found myself absentmindedly picking at the tips. My nails looked worse by the hour, and I ached for someone—anyone—to remove them. More than anything, I longed for fresh air, familiar sounds, and the comfort of my own bed.

On day ten, the doctors said I could go home in two days.

I should've been relieved. But fear crept in again. What if something happened after I left the safety of the machines and professionals?

My hospital room was filled with flowers and cards, love made visible. And yet, I noticed how many rooms around me were empty. Quiet. Unvisited.

The next day, I asked my mom for help. We took the dozens of bouquets I'd received and turned them into smaller arrangements. She picked up miniature vases from a craft store, and together we arranged tiny bouquets of daisies, orchids, and roses.

On day eleven, we wheeled them through the hallways—my mom, Matt, the IV pole, and I delivering flowers to strangers.

Most patients smiled. Some cried. Some spoke.

But each exchange reminded me: within fear, there's room to encourage. Even in my own grief, others still mattered. My heart might have stopped, but it still had purpose.

CHAPTER 9
The Scar on My Chest

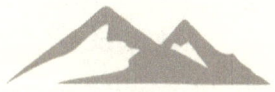

On day twelve, Matt rolled my wheelchair and oxygen tank out of the hospital with three new prescriptions in hand: blood pressure medication, blood thinners, and painkillers that dulled reality's sharp edges. I was also taken off Adderall, which left me even more disconnected in an already fragile state.

In the front seat of Matt's Jeep, I felt relief and anxiousness jostling for space. What if it happened again? Could my heart betray me once more?

Matt gently placed Sadie in my lap. She curled into me, sensing my tension. Her paws hung off of my lap as my hands rested on her back. I could feel her chest rising and falling, and her rapid, strong heartbeat softened my fear. She was alive, and so was I. Sunlight poured through the windshield, a strange comfort after the snowy, desperate drive Matt had made twelve days earlier. Somehow, the warmth held a quiet promise.

Just weeks before, we had been filled with newlywed excitement. Now, the questions hung like storm clouds. Could I ever be that girl again—adventurous, energetic, independent? Would we still be able to start a family?

When we got home, everything felt unfamiliar. Wedding remnants still filled the space: cards, ribbons, stray tissue paper—echoes of a life that already felt distant. All I wanted was a hot shower to rinse off the fear that clung to me like a second skin. The sticky residue from the heart monitor adhesives still marked my chest, leftover reminders of what had just happened. I felt exposed, vulnerable, like I'd been on display for days. No privacy. No pause. I longed to wash it all away—the noise, the monitors, the hands adjusting wires—and retreat into the quiet safety of my mind. Just steam, silence, and the feeling of being whole again in my introverted body.

In the bathroom, I stood naked before the mirror. The bulge of the ICD beneath my skin, the bandages over the incision, and the fine outlines of wires trailing under my flesh—all of it stared back at me. I knew I'd never wear a strapless dress again. A swimsuit would take courage. Tears came, uninvited, as I realized the scar wasn't just physical—it was the silent proof of a war I never chose.

In the shower, the water poured over me, hot and cleansing. I wanted answers. Why me? What now? I didn't have clarity, but I had Matt. His love, steady and unshaken, was like a blanket in a blizzard.

After drying off, he helped me into a simple button-up blouse—no bra, just soft fabric grazing the bandage covering the tender scar. We hooked up the ICD monitor—its blinking lights silently transmitting data to my doctors. Someone, somewhere, was watching. It was meant to reassure me, but instead, it reminded me how vulnerable I'd become.

Before bed, Matt placed the three magnetic monkeys—souvenirs from my hospital stay—on our fridge. The monkeys' cheerful poses made me smile through tears. They became quiet symbols of survival, clinging to the surface just as I clung to hope. I buried my face in Matt's shoulder and cried. Relief. Fear. Gratitude. Terror. All tangled together.

Rebuilding life felt like walking a tightrope—one careful step at a time.

The ICD brought physical and emotional challenges. I couldn't sleep on my stomach or left side—positions I once found restful. I now slept flat on my back, always conscious of its presence under my skin.

Even everyday comfort became a search. Finding a bra that didn't irritate the incision was maddening. After much trial and error, I finally found a soft sleeping bra—the delicate fabric and seamless edges resulted in less rub.

Not long after, Matt and I drove with my parents to retrieve my car from the transportation center, where it had sat untouched since the day everything changed. I wasn't cleared to drive for six months, so Matt would take the wheel.

When we opened the car, a stench rushed out—spoiled steak, vegetables, candy, and a Valentine's card still sealed inside a forgotten grocery bag. The pungency hit hard—a rotten remnant of the life we'd left behind.

I cried—not just from the foul smell, but from the longing to rewind time and erase the events of that day. But as Matt rolled down the windows and the mountain air pushed through, we exchanged a look that said what we both knew: we couldn't go back. We could only move forward together.

Life took on a slower rhythm. Matt returned to work, and I stayed home under my parents' care. Sadie never left my side. She knew when my thoughts turned anxious and would curl close, pressing her warmth into me to melt my fears.

I was drained and far from the physically active woman I'd been. My medication, metoprolol, kept my blood pressure low, but dulled my focus and energy.

During the quiet, I scoured the internet for answers. I searched for survivor stories, medical explanations—anything to help make sense of what had happened. But there was so little out there. Just two organizations: the Sudden Cardiac Arrest Foundation and Parent Heart Watch. Their websites offered comforting summaries, but no in-depth stories, and no real data. The American Heart Association also offered information, though its broader mission focused more on research and stroke. Social media was still new. Online support groups were nonexistent.

I felt completely alone. It would be years before I met another survivor face to face.

In the evenings, Matt came home and filled the space with companionship. To distract ourselves, we turned to Netflix DVDs, devouring episodes of *LOST*. We also revived a shared ritual from our early days: cribbage.

That simple game became a connection to a version of us that felt whole.

It had started years before, during an early spring storm that trapped us indoors. With the ski lifts closed, Matt suggested cribbage—a childhood favorite of his. I fumbled through the rules at first, confused by fifteens and flushes. But Matt was patient, and soon I caught on. Not just caught on—competed fiercely.

We played for hours back then, our laughter filling the small apartment as snow fell outside. Our games revealed our personalities—his quiet strategy balanced by my fiery determination. Every win felt like a minor triumph over the world.

Now, sitting at the kitchen table years later, shuffling that same deck of cards, the joy of those snowbound nights returned. Cribbage wasn't just a game—it was our way of passing time, fueling a little competition, and keeping score in more ways than one. We played countless matches, always teasing each other about who held the upper hand. Eventually, to settle the debate once and for all, we began recording every game in a black, wide-ruled spiral notebook we proudly called *The Lifetime World Series of Cribbage*. We made columns for the date, who had the first deal (since we believed that might tilt the odds), the winner, and a final column to note if someone had been "skunked"—that cruel fate of finishing more than 30 points short of the 121 required to win. By our house rules, the loser had to record the game in the book. Over time, the margins began to hold more than scores: anniversaries, big real estate deals, funny excuses for losing, and the little milestones of our lives at the moment the cards were played. We grew so committed to documenting our rivalry that we even tucked in slips from hotel notepads whenever we traveled, determined not to let a single game go unrecorded.

And in that quiet act of playing cribbage, just Matt, Sadie, and me, I believed that healing wasn't only possible. It had already begun.

CHAPTER 10
Four Life-Changing Words

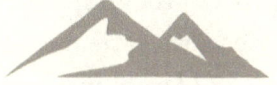

Friends who had traveled for our wedding made the journey again, their presence a balm to my weary soul. Adrienne, my best friend from high school and college, and J., my closest friend since birth, took turns keeping me company during recovery. Their selflessness reminded me that genuine bonds aren't weakened by pain—they're forged in it.

Being with Adrienne brought me back to when we first met. It was the beginning of my junior year in high school. I was working as an office aide, sorting papers at the front desk, when I noticed a pretty girl with brown curly hair in a wine-colored turtleneck and white jean shorts, standing nervously beside her mother. Time slowed as her aura appeared to glow. She looked like she needed a friendly face. I introduced myself with a smile.

"Hi, I'm Lynn."

"I'm Adrienne," she said, soft but curious.

She was a new transfer student from a small private school, and I offered to show her around. After the tour, I invited her to join me for lunch.

"Oh, I'm just going with my mom," she said, unsure.

"It's no trouble," I told her. "I'd love to have lunch with you and introduce you to my friends."

That simple offer marked the beginning of a lifelong friendship. Over time, I came to know Adrienne's story—her mother, who raised her alone through hardship; her estranged father; the devoted grandparents who helped fill the gaps; and the stepfather who eventually became her father. As the eldest of four half-siblings, Adrienne naturally took on a nurturing role in life.

Our connection deepened through spontaneous adventures. From college road trips to Slurpee runs, Adrienne was always up for fun. She embodied everything you could want in a best friend: warm-hearted, energetic, radiant, endlessly optimistic, and unfailingly honest—with just the right amount of hearsay to keep things interesting.

What I treasure most is her loyalty and how effortlessly we fit together. During her visit, we watched TV, caught up on news from Fort Worth, and enjoyed each other's company. Her presence brought the familiar comfort of home, friendship, and assurance that everything would be okay.

Next up was J.

J. was the son of my parents' best friends and had been a steady presence since birth—just sixteen months behind me. He was there for every adventure, celebration, and heartbreak. Even in college, when I pushed everyone away, he once drove hundreds of miles just to sit with me, reminding me that distance would never change our friendship.

During that visit, he shared his truth.

"Lynn, I'm gay," he said, voice trembling with vulnerability.

Over the music, I misheard him and replied casually, "Of course—I know you're J."

He firmly replied. "No, Lynn. I'm gay."

As the words sank in, I felt honored to be the first friend he told. I promised we'd always be close—and that someday, he'd be in my wedding.

But that promise went unfulfilled.

With the opportunity gone, I felt terrible. I told myself binary wedding parties weren't a thing, that Gammy wouldn't have approved, and truthfully, I wasn't sure he'd even make it, deep as he was in his drinking.

Still, none of that erased the guilt. He had shown up. Every time.

Now, as I faced one of the hardest seasons of my life, he was here again. We washed away lingering worries with the last of the wedding champagne, a buzz and laughter softening the ache.

The next day, J. went with me to my first cardiac rehab session.

Surrounded by much older patients, I initially underestimated the challenge. The recumbent bike quickly humbled me—people twice my age pedaled with ease while I struggled to keep up. J. kept things light with his best Rob Schneider impression: *"You can do it!"* His playful commentary helped me laugh through the awkwardness.

Now, in between appointments and recovery, Adrienne and J. weren't just visitors. They were living reminders of who I'd been and the connections that held me up.

As I worked to process the trauma—physical, emotional, and spiritual—the bills arrived.

Each envelope felt like a fresh wound—pages of terms and codes we could barely understand. What was covered? What wasn't? The statements blurred into a mess of line items and jargon that only deepened my sense of frustration.

We were incredibly lucky. The health insurance from my previous work was still active. If my coverage had lapsed during the transition to the Vail Valley Partnership, we would've been financially wrecked. Newly married, with a mortgage and little margin, we could have lost everything. The total cost of care—from the ambulance to the ICD implant—surpassed $1 million. We paid just $5,000.

Even so, the process took its toll. Endless phone calls, paperwork, and efforts to clarify coverage became a second job. Each envelope stirred emotions I was barely holding in.

After eight weeks, I returned to the position I'd barely started before everything changed. What had once been an exciting dream come true, now felt heavy and surreal.

I wasn't just a new employee anymore. I was "the woman who

survived"—the one they'd followed with hushed updates and quiet hope.

Concentrating on any task was exhausting. Basic tasks took more effort than I expected. The drive and energy I'd once prided myself on had vanished. Passion felt out of reach.

Coworkers were kind, but I could feel the distance. Their caution, though well-meaning, felt stifling. I longed to be seen as normal, not fragile, not broken, just capable.

But normal had shifted. Time itself had changed. It no longer felt like a gift—but a ticking clock. "Give it time," people said, over and over.

But when your heart has stopped once, time feels different. It becomes a quiet predator, and every moment is either a blessing or a countdown.

The anxiety lingered. I feared my heart would stop again. The ICD, though life-saving, also tethered me to the worst day of my life. The scar above my chest wasn't just physical—it was psychological. A reminder that the line between life and death was thinner than I'd ever known.

Appointments with Dr. Gaul, our local cardiologist, became routine. The finger-prick blood tests monitored my anticoagulant levels—too low meant risk of clotting, too high meant risk of bleeding.

At the end of each month, Dr. Prager, a kind yet no-nonsense electrophysiologist with a clear, direct manner, traveled from Denver to care for patients in our community. He regularly made these long commutes to rural areas, even as far as Wyoming, providing a lifeline for patients like me, who preferred not to travel hours for specialized care.

His presence highlighted the healthcare disparities between urban and rural communities and the trade-offs we make to live in such a remarkable place. Still, I was deeply grateful for Dr. Prager and his commitment to serving under-resourced populations.

The cardiology clinic's waiting room always made me uneasy. The walls were painted a pale yellow, meant to uplift, but it felt forced, like a fake smile. Posters of Olympic skiers lined the walls—a nod to Dr. Gaul's time as physician for the U.S. Ski Team. These elite athletes had conquered mountains. A drastic contrast to the tension most cardiac patients felt. Most of us were not Olympians. The competitions we faced were invisible, deep within.

A stack of homemade pamphlets caught my eye: *"Dr. Gaul's Guide to Heart Health."* Inside, I expected medical lingo. Instead, I read:

"Eat less. Walk more."

At first, I laughed. That was it? But as I sat there, flipping it over in my hand, I realized the wisdom wasn't in the complexity but in the simplicity.

I already had the eat less part down, but I took the walk more part to heart.

And, I began to walk.

Walking wasn't just movement. It was forward motion and permission to heal, one step at a time.

CHAPTER 11
A Screen of False Promises

Surviving cardiac arrest isn't just a onetime physical trauma—it's a constant acknowledgement of life's unpredictability etched into your psyche. Emerging from the ordeal of cardiac arrest left me with immense gratitude, but it also brought post-traumatic stress disorder (PTSD). Intrusive thoughts, flashbacks, intense emotions, overreacting, irritability, and problems remembering, concentrating, and sleeping were just a few of the symptoms. My thoughts swirled with questions that seemed distant concerns for most people. *What is the meaning of life? What happens when we die? How much time do I have?* The questioning led me to evaluate my existence and confront the whys and hows of my survival.

One conversation at a follow-up appointment left a lasting impression. Dr. Prager stood beside me, explaining the potential causes of my cardiac arrest. It might have been the blood clot, possibly formed during one of our long flights to the islands, or perhaps a side effect of birth control. There was also the possibility that the cardiac arrest itself triggered the clot; no definitive answers could be given. The three major life stressors, or low potassium levels, might have played a role. Or maybe the culprit was an undiagnosed cardiac issue, lying dormant since infancy and finally manifesting in this life-altering event.

Yet despite these possibilities, the exact cause remained a mystery.

It was "idiopathic," a clinical term meaning no specific cause had been found. Yet the literal definition—unknown—felt inadequate to capture the gravity of circumstances and emotions it provoked in me. It was less like a diagnosis and more like a placeholder for uncertainty, fear, and doubt, each layer adding to my growing confusion.

For a while, I accepted the ambiguity. I was grateful to be alive and eager to move forward. But in the quiet moments, I wondered. Was it truly without cause? Or had something been building all along—something invisible to scans and tests?

The medical staff encouraged me to seek therapy to work through the emotional heaviness, and their intentions were kind and earnest.

But I wasn't ready—not yet. The idea of laying my vulnerabilities bare before someone else felt premature. Therapy required readiness; and I had yet to gather the courage to untangle the circumstances and emotions that led to my cardiac arrest.

I had my suspicions about what might have contributed—stress, past lifestyle choices, unresolved inner battles—but these thoughts came as theories, not conclusions. I couldn't share until I first paused to reflect—alone, quietly, honestly.

That's when the memories came—flickering dispatches of another life—vivid and unrelenting. They carried me back to the burden I'd been dragging for years: the influence of false expectations and the relentless pressure to be something I wasn't. That pursuit had shaped much of my life, silently steering my choices and self-worth. I hadn't fully realized how deeply it had cost me—not just physically, but emotionally and spiritually—until now.

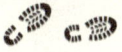

Growing up in the '80s and '90s felt like living in a neon-lit carousel—vibrant, fast-moving, and saturated with the values of consumerism and image. It was a material world, and the pressure to be one of its picture-perfect girls was constant. But deep down, I was cut from a different cloth—earthy, spirited, and a little too wild for the polished boxes others tried to put me in.

The expectation to be proper came from all sides: my sainted Episcopal school, Sunday church services, and perhaps most memorably, my grandparents—Gammy and Papa T. Though they lived in another state, our three or four visits a year left a lasting impression.

Papa T was the second-youngest of eight children, raised in the shadow of the Great Depression. He was the definition of steady—a stoic, honest man whose integrity could've been used to set clocks. His family had established The Wright & Ferguson Funeral Home, one of Mississippi's largest mortuaries. To put himself through business school, he worked overnight shifts there, quietly doing the hard work of picking up the deceased. Only God knows what he must have witnessed in those despicable days of the 1940s. But that's what made Papa T who he was. I was proud to call him my grandfather, especially when he had risen to a position that occasionally drew calls from the President of the United States.

Gammy, his crowning jewel, ran her household with precision, pride, and a little "help." She never held a paying job—except for a single summer scooping ice cream before she married—but her days were full. She maintained a pristine garden, hosted elegant gatherings, and enforced etiquette as if it were a sacred ritual. In her world, elbows stayed off the table, thank-you notes were handwritten, and appearances mattered. She upheld a flawless appearance—meticulously applied makeup, carefully chosen outfits, and a set-and-style helmet hairdo sustained by regular perms and nightly curlers. Polished perfection was her pursuit; she even dyed the veins in her legs when they showed with age.

And yet, beneath the formality, was a quiet, unfaltering love. I still hold tight to golden memories from those visits—the scent of sizzling bacon, hummingbirds flitting outside the window, the comfort of their Southern home. Life with them felt like a step into another time—slower, steadier, beautifully ordered.

At home, my world was equally safe and full of love. My dad, a big-hearted entrepreneur, worked hard to provide not just for our needs, but for our dreams: private school tuition, country club memberships, and the newest gadgets. He was generous, spontaneous, and loyal—always chasing the next big idea. I've often felt the twinkle in his eye was just for me. He saw my fire and, in many ways, recognized himself in it.

My mom was our anchor—calm, faithful, and full of grace. She took us to church, read her Bible, and held our family together through every high and low. When one of my dad's ventures collapsed, she quietly returned to work without complaint, steadying the ship while never letting go of her joy. Mom regularly tuned in to K-LOVE radio station, which played Christian music and talk programs like *Focus on the Family* every time we were in the car. I couldn't stand it. While she absorbed messages about faith and family values, I longed for Guns N' Roses, Madonna, and Michael Jackson. Regardless, she lived the love she believed in quiet, consistent ways.

And then there was Margaret—my older sister and my opposite. She was graceful, dependable, a better fit for the mold our world expected. She exuded a calm I clung to. I often crawled into the extra twin bed in her room just to be near her steady presence. Despite our drop-down, drag-out fights, she always knew when I needed comforting—and she always made me feel better.

One of my earliest memories of that was when I was three. Margaret and I sat side-by-side on a dining room chair, arms wrapped around each other, tears streaming down our cheeks. Outside the window, a truck drove away carrying a black plastic bag. Inside was the body of our beloved dog, Puddy. It was my first real taste of loss—the first time I understood that not everything, or everyone, stays.

Nature and the woods behind our house were my refuge. It was probably only an acre or two of undeveloped land, with a trekked path through trees up a small hill, leading from our terraced backyard to the street behind. But to me, it was a world of exploration. Time was my love language, and if Margaret or my best friend J. weren't available to play, I'd venture out alone, letting my imagination and curiosity guide me.

I'd comb the area for signs of life, hoping to spot baby ducks and raccoons, and hatched elaborate plans to catch them, using laundry baskets, cat food, and a cooler as traps. And sometimes, to my great delight—and my parents' dismay—I was successful.

Anything related to animals, I loved. They offered the kind of acceptance and loyalty I craved—unconditional, wordless, and pure. In a world that sometimes felt confusing and overwhelming, animals understood.

Muffin and PurrPurr were my first genuine attempts at filling that void. I dressed our cats in my baby doll clothes, tucked them into a stroller, and proudly paraded them as if they were my own children. When my next grand idea would bubble up—maybe a costume change or a new game—they'd flee to my mom, silently refusing another of my big plans.

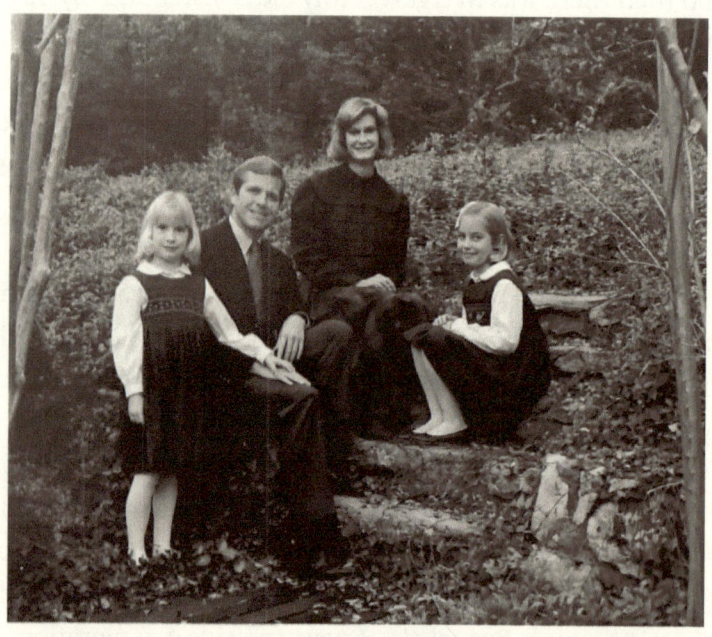

My picture perfect family posing in our terraced yard.

Still, I longed for more furry friends. I didn't want toys or make-believe. I wanted a living, breathing creature to call my own—someone who would choose me back. A pet. A companion. A soul that felt like mine.

In our house, appearances mattered. "Beauty knows no pain," my mom would say as she curled our hair. Margaret thrived in that domain. I, however, bucked against it.

My free spirit made fitting into a polished world difficult. I had a flair for drama and could get what I wanted, whether through negotiation, the occasional tantrum, or a simple smile and flutter of the eyes. My parents' fears about my infant heart condition often gave me an easy out, allowing me to sidestep rules.

Yet beneath the external actions was a deeper, more grounded soul. I longed for connection and authenticity and was relentless in my pursuits. I had an incredible drive to make my desires reality.

My determination often outweighed my caution. Once, to get attention at the pool, I yanked our babysitter's swimsuit top off to make her stop flirting with the lifeguard and pay attention to me. Another time, I struck a deal to endure country club daycare in exchange for my pet hamster, Sam, who became my first real companion.

Then my yearnings led to Teddy Ruxpin. My dad promised to buy me the latest animatronic talking bear if I got an A+ on my spelling test. I did, but when we reached the store, the allure of a small off-white, black and white turn-dial TV captured my interest instead. Dad hesitated, but eventually gave in. That TV became my screen of false expectations. It showed me lavish, beautiful lives and laid the groundwork for chasing fake, unattainable ideals.

As a child, no one realized my mischief pursuits—interrupting conversations, testing boundaries, seeking companions, negotiating deals—weren't just restlessness. They were cries for connection.

In the end, I learned to live by the old mantra: *Try. Try harder. Then try even harder.* Because persistence paid off.

Those early influences and characteristics—my confidence, boldness, and doggedness—were not flaws. They were survival skills. And

I would need every one of them for the journey ahead.

Alongside the essential traits I was developing, a series of major blows would ultimately redirect the trajectory of my life.

Our family had been cruising comfortably. We were living on Easy Street, but there was danger at the door.

The first rupture came on Black Friday, October 13, 1989, when global stock markets plunged in a sudden and devastating crash. My dad, a stockbroker riding the wave of optimism after the more infamous Black Monday of 1987, was caught in the second wreckage. Practically overnight, we lost everything. The fallout was swift and humbling: we relinquished our socialite lifestyle, moved from our beloved home with the forest behind, and the following year we transitioned from our private Christian school to the diverse halls of public school—a shift that marked the beginning of a much different life. As if all that wasn't enough, my beloved furry companion, Sam, also died.

In middle school and high school, I faced setbacks that guided my activities and ultimately brought me here today. I made the cheer squad, then didn't. Too afraid of public failure, I couldn't try out again. Soccer became my new dream, but a routine physical denied my participation because of my heart condition. I returned my first cleats—a pair of purple and black Adidas—with a crushed spirit.

In need of encouragement and purpose, I volunteered at Cook Children's Hospital, the same place that once cared for me, now provided joy. Delivering treats to hurting kids felt like giving back.

The only athletics approved by my doctor were golf and tennis. I chose golf and made it to regionals, but hanging out with friends became my sport.

College followed. I joined Margaret at Texas Tech, pledged Kappa Kappa Gamma, and was voted pledge class president. I thrived, socially and academically, but making the parties was my priority. Along with the good times comes the pressure to perform and conform. And everywhere were messages: be thinner, be prettier, be perfect.

My self-worth eroded slowly. One night, a boyfriend turned violent, striking me and hurling insults that bruised more than just skin. Adrienne rushed to my side, urging me to report the incident. We did. He was expelled, but the damage lingered. I didn't want to be treated this way, but I was. And, on I went, down the road, feeling bad.

Later, Adrienne relayed a cruel comment someone made about my appearance. "He said you look like a beached whale now."

I laughed it off, but the wound was deep. My confidence now crushed under the heaviness of others' judgments.

I stood in front of the mirror, inspecting the changes. The freshman fifteen was real. My once bright eyes now looked puffy. My freckles, another feature I didn't like, glared back at me.

It was shattering my assurance, the quiet comparisons, the feeling of not measuring up. Each morning became a ritual of self-critique, a search for flaws instead of beauty. What started as harmless observations soon fed a deeper discomfort.

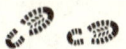

That spring, Papa T passed away from complications of a collapsed lung and a staph infection he acquired while hospitalized. After his death, the family quietly left the hospital. I gave Gammy a hug, but she didn't return it. Gammy wiped a few tears from her cheek, and that was the only visible emotion I witnessed, although I'm sure she cried in private. She was from a generation that had endured more loss than most could imagine, and they had been taught to carry on without complaint.

Gammy had always believed in the power of routine and presentation. Her mantra was simple but steadfast: have a purpose to get up and get dressed every day—even if it was just to go to the grocery store. Grief didn't change that. Each morning after, she still rose early, worked in the garden, then carefully styled her hair, applied her makeup, and selected an outfit that matched both the occasion and her standard. That rhythm of dignity and discipline never wavered. It was her way of holding steady when the rest of life felt uncertain. After years of fulfilling her role as Papa T's wife, she redirected that energy outward, volunteering at a soup kitchen and mentoring women recently released from prison to find work.

She also began mailing me a devotional from her church every few months—thin, hopeful booklets that often went unread. Still, she never forgot. With grandmotherly persistence, she'd call and ask, "Did you read today's message?"

I usually said, "Yes, it was great." But the truth was, I hadn't, and I wasn't interested. Not yet.

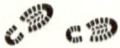

Despite my efforts to regain control through exercise and healthier choices, the pounds stubbornly clung to me. Frustration mounted as I compared myself to others and the images I saw on TV.

I considered the extreme ways others maintained thin figures and tried laxatives, believing it was harmless.

At first, it seemed like a manageable way to control my body. But what began as occasional soon spiraled into more. I reduced my food intake to virtually nothing.

Thinness became the prize. Compliments for my shrinking frame fueled dangerous behaviors. I moved closer to societal ideals, but each step came at a steep and painful cost. I often curled up on the floor with a heating pad, stomach in knots.

By the summer before my senior year, I weighed eighty-five pounds. Friends worried. My sorority sisters staged an intervention. One warned, "You're going to have a heart attack if you don't stop."

Her words haunted me.

My mom finally intervened. On a twilight walk, she turned to me and said, "Lynn, I think you need help."

We visited a behavioral health clinic for eating disorders. I didn't think I belonged there. I told myself I wasn't *that bad*. But I had to admit: my choices had brought me dangerously close to the edge.

Now, years later, after my heart *had* stopped, I understood what they had tried to tell me. My pursuit of perfection, the pain I ignored, the signals I silenced, they all may have led to my current situation.

And in seeing the truth of my past, I found the first threads of healing. I hadn't wanted to admit my intentional suffering, but recognizing it didn't mean sharing it. It meant I could finally accept it and be honest with myself.

The old black-and-white screen had promised me beauty, joy, and success if I just followed the cultural expectations depicted. But it never warned me about the cost.

Now, I was rewiring those influences.

CHAPTER 12
Much Needed Change

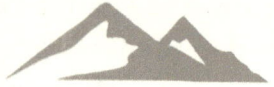

It was the summer of 2002 in Fort Worth, a year after graduating from college, and it was time to break free from the chains I had forged for myself. I wanted to shed my past and embrace the promise of a fresh start. Tired of being stuck, sick, and ready to reclaim my life.

The first step was addressing my struggles head-on. That's when Adderall, an amphetamine prescription drug commonly used to treat attention deficit disorders and narcolepsy, emerged as a possibility. By increasing neurotransmitters like dopamine, it promised improved focus and behavioral control—a potential catalyst for positive change.

Yet, the stigma surrounding its use, often seen as a shortcut for boosting productivity, made me hesitant to try it. Ultimately, I gave it a chance, and the results were transformative. It helped me by shifting my focus, enhancing my perspective, and encouraging regular digestion. But I knew medication alone wasn't enough. I needed a change of scenery, a complete reset.

The mountains of Colorado had been calling me since I was a child, their rugged beauty a symbol of freedom and possibility. It was time to answer that call and begin anew in a place that promised healing and hope.

My parents sold their house in Texas and made the move to Colorado, clearing the way for my transition. With everything I owned stuffed into my car, I pointed north toward the mountains, pursuing the dream of a new life.

I've always been in a hurry, never late, always chasing the next thing, and this time was no different. I couldn't get to Colorado fast enough. It was fitting for my rearview mirror to be small; there wasn't much I wanted to see behind me. But the windshield stretched large and clear, looking ahead to the wide-open future I was desperate to claim.

Two weeks earlier, I had secured my Colorado driver's license, a small rectangle of plastic that served as a symbol for my fresh start. But the rules here were different. In Texas, a speeding ticket was little more than a small fine and a slap on the wrist. In Colorado, every mile over the limit racked up points, and enough points would revoke your license.

Blasting a burned CD labeled "Moving Music," a parting gift from a guy I dated, filled with Widespread Panic and other favorites, I tore through Amarillo by morning, flew across the Oklahoma Panhandle, and raced into Colorado, ignoring every limit sign along the way. As the mountains appeared faintly on the horizon, I exhaled. Freedom.

Then—wew, wew, wew—sirens in my mirror.

My first ticket as an official Colorado resident.

I brushed it off and pressed harder on the gas.

An hour later—more lights, more sirens. Another ticket. Still, I didn't slow down.

Thirty miles from my final destination of Vail, descending from the Eisenhower Tunnel into Silverthorne—wew, wew, wew—a third ticket.

By then, the troopers were expecting me. Word had traveled up the highway: someone was barreling recklessly toward something new, desperate to outrun something old.

With Vail finally in sight—and a stern warning that one more ticket would suspend my brand-new license—I finally lifted my foot from the pedal.

That winter of 2002–03, I eased off in other ways, too: loosening my grip on past obsessions, trusting the road ahead, learning—at last—how to slow down and live again.

For decades, Vail, Colorado, has beckoned adventurers, dreamers, and seekers—people like me. This mountain town, rich in history, is painted with snow-capped peaks that tell stories of resilience and renewal.

Vail is more than a destination; it's a playground of natural grandeur, where the elite rub shoulders with explorers chasing the thrill of the wild. Its global reputation, bolstered by President Ford's family vacation home and its role as a stage for international ski competitions, makes it a magnet for those in search of something extraordinary.

When I first traveled to these mountains at the young age of three, I felt an undeniable sense of connection, as though I was stepping into a legacy that had welcomed countless others before me. Many had come seeking transformation, adventure, or a fresh start—and in that way, I was no different.

Against this magical backdrop, I found my reasons to call Colorado home.

Becoming a ski instructor in Vail would fulfill a lifelong dream, one satisfied out of a desperate need to rediscover the joy and purpose that had eluded me. Vail had always been where my heart felt most alive. Skiing was my passion and the thrill I desired most, and I hoped that returning to the slopes would reignite the spark within me.

To my delight, I was hired to teach children's ski school out of the Lionshead base area. I was proud to wear the blue-on-blue uniforms that bestowed a sense of authority and clout among the visiting guests, though they earned us the unflattering nickname "the Smurfs" from unimpressed ski patrollers.

Yet, the reality of my new role as a ski instructor quickly became apparent. While our uniforms may have conveyed a sense of importance to clueless out-of-towners, they did little to shield me from the less glamorous aspects of instructing the three- to six-year-old program—from wiping away tears and cleaning up spills to tackling bathroom mishaps.

It was an especially exciting time to be in Vail. Early-season storms had brought record snowfall. The ski slopes buzzed with excitement, but it wasn't just the snow that had people talking. The first season of The Bachelorette was airing on ABC, featuring a love story between Vail firefighter Ryan Sutter and the show's star, Trista, unfolding in the very place we called home. Each week, people gathered at bars to watch the latest episode, pointing out familiar landmarks and speculating about the couple's future. There was a sense of shared pride and wonder—that our small mountain town was now part of something magical and widely watched. It felt like we were all part of the story, even if just from the sidelines.

I threw myself into assimilating as a local, determined to leave my Texas roots behind and fully embrace ski town culture. No more standing out as a 'gaper' or awkwardly carrying my skis in ways that turned heads for all the wrong reasons. From now on, I would refrain from saying "y'all," refer to lifts by their numbers, effortlessly navigate the slopes, and remain keenly aware of my presence on the mountain. It was time to blend in, not just as a skier, but as someone who truly belonged.

But Vail wasn't just happy valley—it was layered. For visitors, it was a winter playground of luxury and indulgence, filled with second homes, designer boutiques, and five-star amenities. For locals, it was something different entirely. It was a life of shared adventure, bonded more by passion than privilege. Most of us were just scraping by. It wasn't always easy navigating both worlds, but somewhere between the opulence and the ordinary, I found belonging. Vail's complexities didn't lessen my connection—they deepened it.

I was finally free to be the person I desired to be, liberated from perceptions and past mistakes. Immersed in the enchanting allure of life in a ski town, I felt an undeniable pull to maintain this newfound release and vitality.

Gradually, the shackles of my obsessive habits, forged over years of self-imposed restrictions, were shed. Though remnants of my behaviors lingered—ordering meals without sauce, favoring steamed vegetables, and meticulously scrutinizing every bite—I found myself less engaged in old hangups.

The mountains became my salvation, breathing new life into my weary soul and infusing my spirit with a renewed sense of purpose and belonging. What began as a seasonal sojourn evolved into a steadfast commitment to carve out a life among Colorado's rugged peaks.

With each passing day, my determination to remain in Vail grew stronger. I had arrived seeking solace for a season, but I yearned for the permanence of a lifetime. In the embrace of the mountains, my soul found its home, and I knew that here, among the towering pines and pristine slopes, I was on my way to being my true self.

Securing a summer job was essential if I was staying for the following ski season. That's when I stumbled upon the *Vail Daily* classified ad for an overnight position as resort assistant manager at the Vail Cascade. The opportunity seemed both promising and exciting—a chance to remain in the place I cherished.

The hiring manager, Samantha, was convinced I was the ideal candidate for the job. Perhaps it was our connection as fellow Texans and Kappa Kappa Gamma alums, but more likely, I was the only one who applied. The idea of a twelve-month commitment, though accompanied by grueling hours, was far less daunting than the thought of leaving behind the mountain lifestyle I loved.

As the sun's light faded, a figure walking by the front desk caught my attention. Standing tall, with short dark brown hair, an easy smile, and piercing eyes, he exuded an effortless charm. His athletic build and confident stride hinted at both strength and warmth. Something about his energy captivated me; a glow reminiscent of the day I met Adrienne also illuminated him. A fleeting thought crossed my mind: *I could marry that guy.*

As the evening rush subsided and I took the overnight room service duties, I couldn't help but notice him again—the gentle presence and infectious smile that had already left an impression.

In ski towns like Vail, the men far outnumber the women, probably four to one. There's a saying: "The odds are good, but the goods are odd." I could attest to the truth of that phrase. But this guy was different, he was one of the good ones.

Several weeks later, and unbeknownst to me, Samantha, my hiring manager, had noted our mutual personalities and was determined to play matchmaker. She casually mentioned, "There's this guy in room service who thinks you're cute. His name is Matt."

My cheeks flushed at the prospect, my mind racing with curiosity.

Earlier that day, Samantha approached Matt, informing him, "There's this girl at the front desk who thinks you're really cute and wants to go out with you."

Samantha was orchestrating our introduction behind the scenes.

And so, a romantic dinner beneath a midsummer starlit sky, our love story began.

What started as a casual date quickly evolved into something more meaningful. It was love at first sight, but it didn't stop there. Each encounter brought a growing sense of connection that resonated deeply within me.

Matt had a way of truly seeing me—in ways no one else ever had. He valued my thoughts, even the Southern viewpoints that differed from his New Englander perspectives. He challenged my positions, not to break them down, but to help me grow. With him, I discovered new interpretations and unearthed parts of myself I had never explored before.

We worked hard and played hard, but respectfully. Among Matt's friends, "Sorry I party" was a phrase used half-jokingly to excuse the occasional misstep: one too many cocktails, cutting someone off while skiing, or simply getting lost in laughter and running late. It made sense in every situation, and somehow, it captured the good-times spirit of those younger years.

Still, shadows of the past lingered. My struggles with body image had left scars I feared revealing. What if my imperfections drove him away? I masked my insecurities under the guise of being 'healthy' about food. Matt, ever patient, accepted my quirks without question.

In his steadfastness, I found something extraordinary—a relationship rooted in acceptance. It was as if Matt could see past the walls I had built around myself and chose to love what lay within. His quiet confidence and resolute kindness became a refuge, and with each passing day, my guard came down just a little more.

Mesmerized by his charm, I felt my heart softening in ways I hadn't expected. What started as a spark grew into a steady flame, and for the first time, I let myself imagine a future filled with love, trust, and the kind of partnership I had only dreamed of.

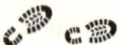

Matt remained my pillar, his loyal presence reminding me I wasn't facing this alone. In the days and months following my cardiac arrest, when fear and uncertainty seemed to lurk around every corner, his relentless support was my salvation. Life with the ICD would never be the same. It was an ever-present reminder of how close I had come to losing everything—and how delicate my recovery could feel.

But Matt's allegiance made all the difference. He didn't attempt to fix everything or push me to move faster than I was ready. Instead, he was there for the insignificant victories: the walks outside, the first night I slept without fear, and even the moments when I broke down under the strain of it all.

With every step forward—no matter how small—I began to see glimmers of hope. Matt's encouragement helped me shift my focus from what I had lost to what I still had: my life, my family, and the chance to write a new future. His patience and love helped find the way, one day at a time, through the uncertainty of our new reality.

CHAPTER 13
Am I The Only One Questioning?

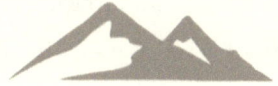

Experiencing a brush with death inevitably prompts a complex reflection on life's purpose and the existence of something greater than ourselves. In the wake of my near-death incident, Matt and I felt compelled to explore spirituality more deeply, attending services at The Vail Church regularly of our own accord, not just as a formality tied to our marriage.

That decision marked the beginning of a transformative journey. From the moment we stepped through the doors, we were welcomed by an accepting and encouraging community.

Their generosity knew no bounds. People from the church had already provided meals, helped with tasks, and offered heartfelt prayers for both our marriage and my recovery.

With youthful charisma and a disarming presence, Pastor Craig quickly became central to our spiritual perspectives. His unique blend of humor and insight made each lesson both engaging and thought-provoking, inviting us to wrestle with life's deeper questions.

Like many pastors, he had a few go-to one-liners that stuck with you. "Don't be a jerk for Jesus," he reminded us that too often, well-intentioned believers alienate others by policing instead of accepting.

"We're all failing forward" was his mantra: after our mid-twenties, our bodies begin to decline—now failing yet still enduring and moving toward complete failure.

And perhaps his most sobering line: "The best odds in the world—one out of one will die."

That stark truth had haunted me. But as I listened to him teach on Sunday mornings and spent time in quiet reflection, death began to lose its sting. It became less of a fear and more of a motivator to live with purpose.

Through Pastor Craig's guidance, we weren't just absorbing ideas. We were being moved—challenged, inspired, and changed. His words did more than inform; they provoked and ultimately inspired us to become better people by believing in something greater than ourselves.

With our attendance regular and my health stable, Pastor Craig approached us with a bold request: "Your story is powerful. Would you be willing to share your testimony one Sunday morning?"

My heart sank. I smiled politely and nodded noncommittally, but inside, I was flooded with apprehension. A testimony? That word alone felt loaded. I was expected to offer some nice, neatly tied story declaring faith. But my reality was far messier.

The truth was, certainty eluded me. Questions—big ones—about God, suffering, and the meaning of it all stirred beneath the surface. I hadn't reached the firm conviction I thought was necessary to speak publicly about beliefs. Instead of confidence, I feared revealing the cracks.

Was I the only one who sat in the rows unsure, the only one on an honest search?

Beneath the questioning was a quieter nudge to step up and be real. Though still uncertain about the details of our relationship with God, we felt compelled to say yes. After all, our story, shaped by survival and the search for meaning, might offer hope to someone.

That invitation sparked a new level of introspection. *Why was my life saved? Where was I meant to go from here?*

I realized that finding purpose had to begin with gratitude. That summer, I turned my focus to the individuals who had saved my life. It was time to thank them—not just in words, but in a way that felt meaningful.

With support from my Texas family, we organized a proper Lone Star-style BBQ brisket feast for the first responders. It wasn't just a thank-you; it was a step toward understanding.

Meeting with the paramedics gave me a chance to hear the incident from their perspective. They shared that most cardiac arrest calls didn't end well, which made my survival especially remarkable.

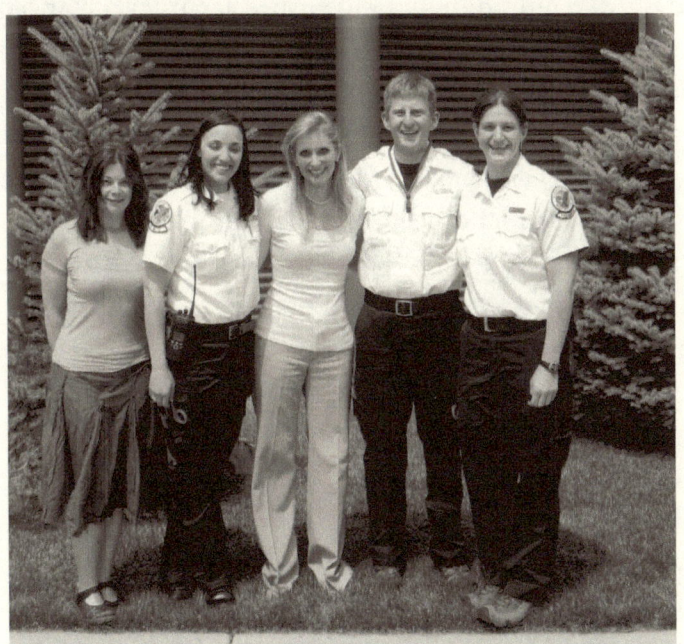

Responding paramedics, Maura, Jenn, me, Graham, and Dawn.

As I listened, I realized every person involved had played a role in keeping me alive. One responder even shared how the experience of saving my life had changed hers by inspiring her to continue with the profession and pursue further education.

That moment crystallized something: surviving wasn't just my turning point, it was also a defining moment for others.

Still, a lingering question remained: What does it all mean if life can end so abruptly?

In the months that followed, I struggled to find my footing at the Vail Valley Partnership. Moving to a new office in the town nearby offered some distance from the scene of my cardiac arrest, but it wasn't enough to clear the fog. The beta-blockers left me sluggish, my blood pressure already low. The time I spent without oxygen had dulled my cognitive sharpness, and fatigue became a constant companion. As soon as I returned home from work, I'd want to climb right into bed.

Responses which should be second nature, such as identifying left and right, required thought to ensure accuracy. I glanced down at my hands to see which thumb and index fingers made the shape of an L. I was desperate for an increase in energy and focus

Despite the caution about Adderall, I needed clarity. Eventually, I returned to my general practitioner to request a prescription renewal. When he asked how I'd been, I explained my cardiac arrest and current state.

What happened next surprised me. He casually referred to my event as a "heart attack."

"Cardiac arrest," I firmly corrected.

He dismissed it. "Oh, same thing."

But they aren't the same—not even close. A heart attack is a plumbing problem: a blockage in the arteries. Cardiac arrest is electrical: an energy failure. The difference is more than technical—it's the difference between alive and breathing and instant death.

That moment stuck with me. If even a licensed doctor could confuse the two, how much awareness was still needed?

Aside from the unsettling exchange, he authorized my prescription. I left with a renewed focus—but also a deeper appreciation for how misunderstood cardiac arrest is.

Meanwhile, the gratitude I felt toward those who had saved me was overwhelming—and oddly paralyzing. What do you say? How can you repay someone for saving your life?

As I continued working at the Vail Valley Partnership, it became clear the position had served its purpose. The timing, the CPR, the location—it all felt too precise to be a coincidence.

Everything had lined up to make my survival possible, yet every single detail was outside of my control.

But that moment had passed. The job no longer held meaning. It was time to go.

When the opportunity came to help my dad with one of his business ventures, I didn't hesitate. It felt like the right step—a way to move forward and leave the trauma behind.

I walked away carrying not just the memory of survival, but the freedom to build a new life. One defined not by what had happened, but by what came next.

CHAPTER 14
The Two Most Pivotal Gifts

As the winter months approached once again, I eagerly anticipated returning to one of my greatest passions—skiing. On a radiant blue-sky day at Vail Mountain, my ever-watchful mom and I headed to Golden Peak for my first time back on the slopes. Yet an unexpected encounter reminded me how fortunate I was.

As we walked through the lodge at the base of the mountain, I caught sight of a group of Wounded Warriors, most of them amputees from their service in Afghanistan, gearing up for an adaptive ski program. My enthusiasm plummeted. And my pace slowed. The unfiltered courage etched on their faces brought a lump to my throat, and tears blurred my vision.

In that powerful moment, I was struck by the truth that I could hardly speak aloud. Turning to my mom, I whispered, "That could have been me."

I imagined what life would look like if they had taken my leg. Would I still hike or ski the mountains I loved? Would I have had the courage to continue?

Maybe I would've found even more determination—driven not just by survival, but by the public reminder of what I had lost. Or maybe the grief and limitation would have made showing up feel impossible.

But I didn't lose my leg. And somehow, that made me feel both fortunate and responsible. The ability to move freely, to stand in front of others—these weren't small things. They were gifts. Gifts that meant I had a duty to walk with purpose.

The thought of losing my leg just ten months earlier overwhelmed me—but also stirred reverence. Reverence for the resilience of the human body. Reverence for the unbreakable human spirit. Deep down, I knew if I had lost my leg, I might not have found the strength to carry on.

That moment revealed a deeper truth: maybe life never gives us more than we can endure.

As I stood there, reflecting on the life I had narrowly avoided, I was in awe of the strength that saved my leg. I realized I was never truly alone. Even when I couldn't see it, a higher help was over it all.

I didn't know then that having the ability to walk would change my life—but it would, in ways I couldn't yet imagine. And it was only possible because I still had both of my legs—two gifts I would never again take for granted.

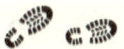

As the anniversary of my cardiac arrest approached, I was awash in emotion. The American Heart Association (AHA) prepared to present the Heartsaver Hero Award—an acknowledgment of the courageous individuals whose quick actions, administering CPR and defibrillation, had saved my life.

The ceremony became a moving tribute to life and gratitude. A chance to honor the bystanders, firefighters, and paramedics who had acted so swiftly and selflessly. The unsung heroes who risk everything to protect the lives of strangers.

Among them was Sue Froeschle, the citizen responder from the Vail Valley Partnership who had performed CPR. As we reunited, she shared a vivid memory of that fateful day.

"You sure look better than last Valentine's Day," she joked warmly.

As a gesture of kindness, Sue handed me a small wooden jewelry box. Inside lay a delicate gold and ruby heart necklace—a cherished gift from her husband.

"He said I don't wear it much," she explained. "And I wanted you to have it."

I was overcome with emotion. The necklace wasn't just a gift—it was a sacred symbol of her role in my survival. I removed it from the box, and Sue gently fastened it around my neck. A piece of her heart now rested near mine.

I wanted to express my gratitude in return, in a way that words alone couldn't capture. I created a handmade Valentine. Carefully, I placed eight photos—images that held deep meaning: snapshots of life, joy, and second chances from the past year. Alongside the pictures, I brought flowers and treats, a humble offering for the people who had saved my life.

Their actions had changed my world forever, and they deserved to know.

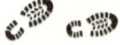

At last, the grip of a cold, dark year loosened. Nature signaled the shift. Birds chirped in harmony. The trees blossomed with color and promise. The seasons were changing, and something within me stirred.

With the arrival of spring, my strength slowly returned. I grew restless within the confines of recovery. My short walks weren't enough anymore. I needed air, space, movement—proof that I was alive.

And what began as walking soon turned into hiking.

Our neighborhood is nestled between rugged mountains where the Eagle River divides the valley floor. Just up the road from our townhouse, a newly cleared trail wound its way into the White River National Forest.

To reach the trailhead, I climbed a quarter-mile stretch of road, past the golf course, and through a gap in the fence. I paused there, my breath coming harder than expected. The incline ahead seemed daunting. I was still in cardiac rehabilitation. I wasn't yet the hiker I had once been.

But I pressed forward, one slow, determined step at a time.

At the trail's fork, I turned west, where the incline eased. Beneath towering pines and newly budding aspens, I found my rhythm again. My lungs filled with crisp mountain air. My legs carried me farther than I thought possible.

There was no grand epiphany or lightning bolt from above on that hike. But something in me shifted. I felt alive. I felt well. I felt at home.

The path forward had begun with a simple pamphlet in a waiting room. Its quiet message was: "Eat less. Walk more." It sounded so ordinary, almost trite. But walking, I discovered, wasn't just physical therapy. It was spiritual therapy—a reminder that even fragile hearts can find their way forward, with one foot in front of the other.

PART 2

A Changed Heart
Life After Cardiac Arrest

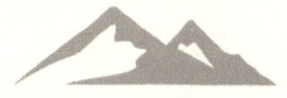

CHAPTER 15
Hidden Connections

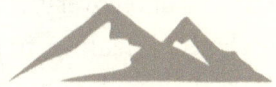

Hiking the trail behind our house became a ritual; a sacred time to connect with nature, myself, and the universe. Rain, snow, or shine, I resolved to keep walking. Restoring my strength wasn't just physical—it was mental—mending the unseen wounds.

With each hike, I explored the trail and my life. The steady rhythm of my footsteps became meditation, slowly unraveling the choices and moments that had brought me to that pivotal event. The towering trees and flowing river mirrored my journey—their resilience a quiet testament to survival against adversity.

I began to make sense of my past—childhood joys, adolescent struggles, self-inflicted wounds, and moments of redemption. Each recollection felt like a trail marker—reminding me of who I used to be, while pointing toward the stronger, more grounded person I was becoming.

I came to understand that sharing my story meant confronting it fully. The choices I had made, the roads I had taken—all played a role in the events that led to my cardiac arrest.

As I walked, questions swirled in my mind: What is the purpose of this life? What lies beyond our earthly perceptions? Deep in the heart of the wilderness, I found tranquility and clarity in the stillness of the trees and the sweep of the sky.

Nature became my confidant, offering quiet wisdom I hadn't found elsewhere. The river carving its path through stone, wildflowers blooming in rocky soil—all of it reflected my effort to find beauty and meaning in the aftermath of trauma.

Every detail, from the towering peaks to the faint hum of wind threading through the valley, whispered of fragile life.

Walking wasn't just a means of recovery; it was a declaration. Each step and hike brought me closer to healing, to purpose, to possibility.

With every step, I became more convinced that I was saved for something significant and unique, though I didn't yet know what that was.

My innermost being was confident: I had been spared to save others.

Every element of February 14 seemed connected, as if guided by an unseen hand: the intuitive pull to accept the job, the office's proximity to the fire station, Sue's swift and decisive CPR. Each detail aligned perfectly, culminating in that singular, lifesaving moment. While some might call it fate or luck, I believed it was part of something greater—like divine timing or a purpose only God could orchestrate.

Just as an aspen tree along the trail appears to stand alone, my cardiac arrest once felt like a solitary incident. But like the aspen grove, where every tree is rooted in one interconnected system beneath the surface, I saw how that moment was connected to something much larger—a web of people, timing, and purpose. What looked isolated was, in truth, deeply entwined. And so was my survival.

The circumstances that saved my life weren't random. They were tightly interwoven events, guided by something more extraordinary than I could comprehend.

But before I could fulfill any convictions, I had to find the strength to learn to live again.

One of the most significant challenges that comes with surviving is coping with the PTSD and anxieties that follow. Living with a "broken heart" is both obtrusive and perpetual. Though the physical scars were hidden beneath my clothing, the psychological wounds remained painful and ever-present.

The trauma of that day would linger, emblazoned in my being. It resurfaced during moments of fear and uncertainty, gripping me with the thought: *Will this be the day my heart finally stops for good?* Even in moments of joy or peace, that heaviness never fully lifts. The fragility of life, once distant and abstract, had become a constant companion.

But the emotional toll wasn't the only challenge. The brain fog continued—a quiet, relentless struggle. Tasks that had once felt effortless now required added energy: remembering names, following conversations. My brain needed extra time to "lift off." The fight wasn't visible, but it was there.

I became more introverted than ever before. Cognitive blips were frequent, and I started internalizing everything before speaking. But the more I overthought, the more my words tangled—if they came out at all. Often, I stayed silent, even when what I wanted to say felt deeply important.

Surviving a near-death experience isn't a single victory—it's a daily battle. Fear creeps in, but I learned to take each thought captive and replace it with gratitude and resolve. Overcoming required a new way of living—a new perspective.

The trail became my temple—a place where I could confront past and present challenges head-on. With every walk, I leaned into the process of living, one foot in front of the other. The seasons and terrain might change, but my commitment to keep moving forward wouldn't waver.

I was coming to understand that life's greatest gifts often emerge from its hardest trials. The paths we tread—no matter how rocky the road or heavy the load—shape us. For me, every climb along that trail, through pain and toward purpose, was leading me to exactly where I needed to be.

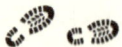

STEP TO REDUCE ANXIETY AND INCREASE HEART HOPE:

Get outside and move. Sunshine, fresh air, and motion shift your mindset and bring clarity.

CHAPTER 16
Ascending From the Valley

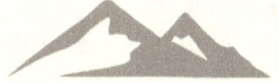

Cool morning air brushed against my face as I buckled my pack. Ahead, the trail climbed steeply, winding through a dense forest that seemed to close in with every step. The last ascent had been daunting, and for a moment, when the path finally leveled out, I thought I had reached the top. But just beyond the clearing, another hill rose into view—just when you think you've made it through, a new challenge appears.

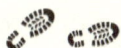

On September 15, 2008, the financial world was rocked by the collapse of Lehman Brothers, marking the beginning of the global economic crisis. As the fourth-largest U.S. investment firm, Lehman's entanglement in mortgage-backed securities left it vulnerable to the housing market's decline. The shockwaves reached every corner of the country, including ours.

For Matt, a rising realtor, the impact was immediate and profound. The downfall struck at the core of his profession. In the quiet comfort of the Vail Valley, the crisis initially seemed far away. But its devastation was undeniable when the tidal wave of foreclosures and job losses finally swept in.

The downturn hit every layer of life. The once-thriving housing market imploded, leaving homeowners with underwater properties and uncertain futures. Ours was no exception. We had recently purchased our home for $485,000. Now, it was worth only $275,000.

Our mortgage was upside down—we owed more than the house was worth—but we stayed the course. Every dollar mattered. Matt took whatever work he could find in a dwindling industry, while my steady paycheck became our financial crutch.

As one year turned into two, my life post-cardiac arrest was feeling strangely routine. But I felt a yearning deep within me—a longing to nurture, to find joy beyond survival. That instinct led to one of the most impulsive, and arguably disrespectful, decisions I made in our marriage: I brought home a second dog.

It began as a spontaneous adventure. Samantha, my old boss and the friend who introduced me to Matt, was swimming in a race at Horsetooth Reservoir. Coincidentally, the breeder who'd given us Sadie lived nearby.

Samantha recruited me to kayak beside her for safety. I had zero paddling skills, but she assured me I could do it. As I clumsily paddled across the water beside seasoned athletes, I couldn't shake my ulterior motive. After the race, we visited the breeder, and two twelve-week-old Blenheim puppies tumbled out to greet us. One, in particular, captured my heart.

We made a list of pros and cons, and I convinced myself it was in our best interest. Samantha promised to take the puppy if Matt didn't want him. That was enough justification for me. I wrote the check and brought him home.

Matt and Sadie were curled up on the couch when I arrived, enjoying a peaceful afternoon. Their relaxation ended the moment I walked in. Matt's face was a mix of confusion and disbelief.

"How could you make this decision without me?" he disappointedly asked—a tone I rarely heard from him.

He called his parents in frustration. Their reply? "Matt, if she wants a dog that bad, let her have one."

I burst into tears and took the puppy to Samantha's house. But by the time I returned home, Matt had changed his mind. "Go get him," he said.

When my parents visited, my mom noticed the little brown mark shaped like lips near his snout. "It looks like God kissed him and told him to make someone happy," she said. And that's exactly what he did.

Aside from the bumpy start, Charlie—later nicknamed Chaz-Monkey-Poo-Poo—became part of the family. Matt, who had initially resisted, soon formed a bond with him that surpassed all expectations. Sadie only tolerated him.

One quiet evening not long after, Matt and I played cribbage on the deck, sipping wine while the dogs napped between us. The stars appeared in the night sky.

"Do you ever think about what comes next?" I asked, surprising even myself with the question.

Matt glanced at me, then looked back toward the horizon. "You mean work? Life? Kids?"

"All of it," I said. "Sometimes I feel like we've been surviving for so long . . . . I don't know what thriving even looks like anymore."

He nodded slowly. "I still want to build something real. A successful career. But I also want a family. Maybe we're ready?"

I looked down at Charlie, his head nestled on my lap. "Yeah, I think I'm ready. Let's dream about our future again."

That night, we didn't make a plan. But we made a quiet agreement: to reach for something more than recovery—to chase life together, whatever it brought.

Looking back, I realize the toll the puppy decision took on Matt. It wasn't just about a dog—it was about respect and partnership. Still, Charlie's joy-filled spirit brought a lightness we didn't know we were missing.

As much as we loved Charlie, a puppy wouldn't fulfill the more instinctive desire in my heart. By early 2010, we felt ready to try for a child.

My cardiac arrest still reigned over our decisions, but I'd grown comfortable living with my ICD, and years with no problems had built my confidence.

We consulted my electrophysiologist, Dr. Prager. Sitting in that familiar office surrounded by beeping monitors and ICD interrogation machines, I felt the immensity of the moment. When he gave us the green light, it was as if a door to our previous lives had opened.

We tossed the birth control and got to work.

Soon, two pink lines on a pregnancy test sent us into joyful disbelief. We were going to be parents.

At our first ultrasound, we held our breath as the black-and-white screen flickered to life—a tiny heartbeat. We were overcome with hope.

Because of my medical history, I was high-risk and referred to a specialist in Denver. Matt stayed behind to work while my dad drove me to the appointment.

The technician's silence during the scan made my stomach sink. She stepped out to speak with the doctor. When they returned, the news was devastating: the baby's heart had stopped.

Numb, I agreed to a procedure to remove what was left. My dad drove me home as I stared out the window, stunned by grief.

When I called to inform Matt, his voice cracked with sorrow. We had dared to hope. Now we had to let go.

My mom's reaction shocked me. "God will use this for good," she said.

To me, it was salt in the wound, a painful blow to my already questionable faith. How could God, in all His "goodness," allow me to endure the trauma of cardiac arrest, only to heap another layer of suffering upon me?

Hadn't I already borne more than my fair share of pain and adversity? However, my past suffering didn't make me immune to more challenges.

The notion that our miscarriage could be part of some sacred plan seemed unfathomable, if not downright cruel. Finding meaning in our loss felt like an impossible task.

I lashed out at her, unable to accept her words. I wasn't ready to find purpose in this pain.

The days that followed were heavy. We had already shared the news of the pregnancy with loved ones. Now, we had to tell them we had lost it.

Matt canceled a long-awaited ski trip to stay home with me. The procedure left me cramping, bleeding, and full of sorrow.

Miscarriage is a lonely grief. It's full of questions—what did I do wrong? Could I have prevented this? But it's not a failure. It's more common than we realize, affecting one in five pregnancies. The encouraging statistic, most go on to have healthy babies. Still, healing and conceiving take time.

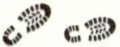

Soon after, I traveled to see Gammy in Jackson, Mississippi. I was still bleeding, but my doctor cleared the trip. Gammy, my only living grandparent, welcomed me with love and her usual spoiling.

I had planned to shop for nursery fabric. Instead, Gammy, never one to hold back, pointed to the scowl line between my eyebrows. "Let's go see my dermatologist," she said, offering Botox as a gift.

Vanity had long been a struggle for me. Cultural expectations, family ideals, and social influences had all played a role in my insecurities. Beauty had always seemed synonymous with worth. My battle with an eating disorder displayed the lengths to which I had gone in pursuit of the elusive standards.

Though I accepted her gift, I recognized what it represented—not just appearance but pressure to conform.

Gammy also opened up about her stillbirth. I couldn't imagine losing a full-term baby. Her experience put my pain into perspective.

I returned home with a softer heart and forehead, and the freshness of my pain beginning to dull.

My mom's words no longer stung as they once had. Maybe, just maybe, something beautiful could come from the sorrow.

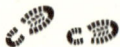

STEP TO REDUCE ANXIETY AND INCREASE HEART HOPE:

Don't expect easy. Even dark seasons hold meaning and shape what's coming.

CHAPTER 17
Mountain of Purpose

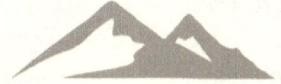

Matt's college friend Ben and his wife Chelsey had become close friends. Now living in Denver and weekend warriors, they frequently made the two-hour trip to Vail, and hosting them in our spare bedroom revived our vibrant social lives—double-dates and slope-side adventures.

Their routine was set—they would drive up to the mountains on Friday evenings and stay until Sunday. Ski dates, followed by après-ski gatherings and cozy dinners by the fire, became our cherished tradition.

Chelsey, with her ambition and compassion, offered understanding as I continued navigating the challenges of living with a cardiac condition. My situation resonated with her—her father had suffered from similar health issues, and she had cardiovascular complications in her youth. We continued to grow closer through shared experiences and mutual support.

We also reveled in challenging ourselves to keep up with Matt and Ben on the most difficult runs. On one particular bluebird day, Chelsey and I took a different route from the boys. The detour felt like a slight relief—a girls' adventure. I darted around a mogul, clipped a hard patch of snow, and tumbled. It seemed minor, and I popped up quickly.

"Lynn, you all right?" she asked, concerned.

"Yeah! I'm great, Chels. Let's go!" I replied, brushing it off with a laugh.

A few weeks later, after a ski day and après at Vendetta's, the local pizza joint and ski patrol hangout, I struggled to breathe while climbing stairs at the transportation center. Panic gripped me, and Chelsey, quick to respond, handed me a paper bag to slow my breathing.

In the days that followed, a strange rhythmic ticking sensation emerged in my left arm, faint pulses near the vicinity of my ICD. I tried to ignore them, but the unease grew.

Eventually, I scheduled an appointment with Dr. Prager. After interrogating my device, he found a lead fracture that occurred at the precise day and time as that ski fall with Chelsey. Fortunately, it was the atrial lead, which was less critical in my case. We scheduled surgery to fix it after ski season. Since my battery was also nearing depletion, I requested a replacement during the procedure and asked if I could keep the old device as a memento. They agreed to both.

The procedure was routine and uneventful. My medical team accessed the original incision, added a new lead, and swapped out the old ICD. I was home within twenty-four hours, my chest sore but my spirit intact. I returned to normalcy within a few weeks.

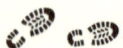

Later that summer, Chelsey encouraged me to share my story with Young Hearts, a Denver-based group of twenty- and thirty-year-olds supporting the AHA. I hesitated, but her conviction persuaded me.

Matt and I drove to Denver, my heart pounding with anticipation. As I stood before the audience and recounted February 14, 2007, a tingle of liberation rushed through me. The words flowed nervously, yet I hoped my story held the potential to inspire and uplift others. The vulnerability was worth it.

Still, after the applause faded, I slipped quietly to the side, unsure how to process the attention. Public speaking didn't come naturally to me. I had always preferred the safety of behind-the-scenes work—the quiet support roles, the creative spaces. Being the one in front made me feel exposed. But something was shifting. I realized that sharing my experience wasn't about seeking recognition—it was about awareness and providing others with information that could save lives.

Chelsey's mother, Trisha, an AHA advocate, attended and recognized the transformative power of my story and encouraged me to use it more broadly. Her support ignited something within me. I realized that this ordeal—this survival—had purpose.

We all became more involved with the AHA, attending the Heart Walk, Heart Ball, Go Red for Women Luncheon, and other events. It felt good to acknowledge the importance of their work that saves lives, just like mine.

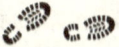

While involvement with the AHA was fulfilling, they didn't have a local office, and my desire to make tangible change grew stronger. I realized that to reach the summit, I needed a solid understanding of the actions required to help someone in cardiac arrest.

I rallied Matt, my mom, and Samantha to take an AHA CPR/First Aid certification course with me. The eight-hour in-person training was intense. The nuances—ratios, techniques, age adjustments—overwhelmed me. Though certified, I left uncertain I'd recall it in a crisis.

I thought about Sue, who performed my chest compressions, and the prepared confidence she showed. I knew I had to do more than pass a test—I needed to simplify the message to reach more people. While some had training through jobs, most would be discouraged by long sessions and costs. I realized that true competence in CPR required a relatable message and regular practice. I felt driven to address the issue.

In the car afterward, I ranted to Matt, "We graduated from high school and college, and no one taught us this. If we'd been on our honeymoon, you wouldn't have known what to do. I wouldn't be alive. Why isn't this basic education? Where can you even find a defibrillator?"

That conversation was a turning point. My voice was determined and firm: "People need this. I want to teach CPR. I'm going to become an instructor."

The very next week, I started researching the qualifications.

My mom was simultaneously preparing to launch Heart Hope, her nonprofit, to provide spiritual encouragement. Samantha was developing a women's health initiative in Ghana. Their boldness inspired me. Why not me? Saving lives could be my personal mission.

I kept thinking about the people who didn't survive cardiac arrest because no one knew what to do. I thought about the terrifying silence of that moment—how close I came to being one of them—and how ninety percent never get a second chance.

It wasn't enough to just be grateful anymore. I needed to *do* something. The calling I felt wasn't just professional—it was emotional. It was spiritual. I benefited from what preparedness looked like through Sue, and I'd seen what hesitation looked like in Matt. I had lived the outcome.

More than once, I asked myself, *Why did I survive? Why me?*

And though the answers didn't come easily, one truth rose to the surface: survival is a gift—but also a responsibility. I couldn't just return to "normal." Something had to change. I had to be part of that change.

So, when my dad's company offered voluntary layoffs, I saw an opening. It felt reckless and right all at once. And I knew this wasn't just about me anymore. It was about the lives I might help save.

Inspired to broach the subject as we watched an episode of *What Would You Do?* with John Quinones, I turned to Matt: "Would people know what to do if they witnessed a cardiac arrest?" I asked, recalling Matt's admission that he wouldn't have been prepared on that Valentine's Day in 2007.

"Yeah, I'm not sure. Probably not most," he replied with uncertainty.

I unveiled my plan to start a nonprofit to teach CPR and place defibrillators—free, accessible, lifesaving education and resources.

He hesitated. "As a hobby, or . . . ?"

I explained, "I don't know. But I feel this is why my life was saved—to save others. Let's just see what happens. We'll try it. If we can't maintain, I'll get a job."

He paused, then nodded. "Okay. What's next?"

I filed for nonprofit status, learning as I went. My mom's recent application helped with the IRS forms. I built a brand: Starting Hearts. Our logo featured arms forming the V of a heart with stacked CPR hands at the bottom, and a lightning bolt to represent the importance of defibrillation. Our tagline: "Anyone. Anywhere. Anytime. Are YOU ready?"

The problem was obvious. Too many people died because the public didn't know what to do. Famous figures like Michael Jackson and Frank Sinatra were lost to cardiac arrest. Most of these stories were mislabeled or misunderstood. I wanted to change that.

The mission was becoming more than training—it was about reframing cardiac arrest in public consciousness.

That summer, I applied for jobs half-heartedly but knew I was working towards a higher position. My focus shifted from what I had lost to what I could build.

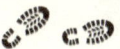

With no official job to report to, my mother encouraged me to attend a women's Bible study called "Cracked Pots." Upon hearing the name, I chuckled, "Crackpots? What sort of study is this, Mom?"

The title made me laugh, but the story it referenced—about a flawed pot that, through its fracture, watered flowers along a path—was touching. I saw how my cracks could lead to beauty.

I didn't expect to connect with anyone there, but I noticed a beautiful girl about my age. After the lesson, she introduced herself. "Hi, I saw you sitting across the room. My name is Rachel."

That simple gesture made me feel welcome and interested in coming back. We both attended the rest of the summer. Rachel continued to be a positive influence by making CDs of inspirational music and encouraging us to read books like "What's It Like to Be Married to Me?" an honest reflection that challenged us to become better wives.

I also started reading a Bible my mom gave me—365 Days of Scripture—designed to be completed in one year.

Each day typically included two chapters of a book, a passage from Proverbs, and one from the Psalms. To my surprise, the readings were transformative. It answered questions I didn't even know I had. As I continued, I understood why the Bible is the best-selling book and most enduring narrative of all time. It wasn't just ancient text. It was relevant. And it was speaking to me.

Soon after, I took the K-LOVE challenge: thirty days of only Christian music. It transformed my mindset. "Worship music" had changed, no longer just the hymns my mom once played—it spanned from country to rap to hard rock, but with lyrics that were encouraging. Matt and I still listened to the classics and cultural music of the day, but when I was alone, I turned to this new genre. It also became my favorite part of going to church.

Religion had always been my mom's thing—not mine. With prayer, I wasn't sure what to do. I didn't have the words, so I just sent up a thought and hoped it was heard:

"God, I do not know who you are, what you are, or where to even begin—but I'm trusting you exist. If this is what you want for my life, I don't know what comes next, but I'm believing you'll make a way."

Even though I was pursuing something deeper spiritually, I rarely talked about it. I've spent much of my life trying to be liked, to keep the peace, and to avoid offending anyone. Belief in God is the most polarizing subject around.

Unless I knew someone held similar beliefs, I refrained from speaking of my quest. Most of our friends identified as agnostic or atheist, so I avoided revealing any convictions. Some might have known we were going to church, but I would play it down by saying, "Well, you don't survive a near-death experience without a 'meet your Maker' moment," and leave it at that. It's easier than opening the door to misunderstanding or judgment.

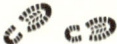

Around this time, I attended the Vail Valley Breast Cancer Awareness Group luncheon, where Robin Roberts spoke about her memoir. Watching Brenda Himelfarb, the group's founder, gave me hope that Starting Hearts could someday thrive as her organization had. But Robin's words struck deep: "Make your mess your message."

That line changed everything. I realized Starting Hearts wasn't just a nonprofit. It was my message. My mess—my cardiac arrest, my struggles, my survival—wasn't just for me. It could save others.

Rarely do you find passion in your opportunities and skills; you find it in your hurts and scars.

And in pouring my energy into that cause, I found some relief from the ache of waiting for a child.

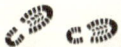

Later that summer, I ran into Sue Froeschle, the woman who had performed CPR on me years before, at the local farmer's market. I shared my plans for Starting Hearts.

Without hesitation, she pulled out a twenty-dollar bill—our first donation. It wasn't about the money. It was confirmation. A moment

I'd never forget.

That Labor Day, my childhood friend J. came to visit. Newly sober, he glowed with clarity and peace. A refined sense of presence accompanied his newfound dependability, energy, and eloquence. His carefree laugh reminded me of when we were kids. I admired his commitment.

We hiked Beaver Lake Trail, and I struggled to catch my breath. The air felt thin, and my pulse felt faint.

"Lynn, are you alright?" J. inquired, the second person within a few weeks to ask me that.

"I don't know," I admitted. "I just need to sit down."

I made it home, but soon realized something was wrong. My heart rate was barely thirty beats per minute. My ICD paced at 65, so it clearly wasn't working.

I was transported by ambulance to a medical center outside of Denver to determine the cause. Once again, Matt hastily packed up the car and followed the ambulance down I-70. The situation's urgency pressed down on us as we traveled separately, unsure of what lay ahead.

Once there, the doctor on duty quickly performed an operation to determine the source of the problem. During the ICD replacement several months before, one lead had been loosely secured. With one simple screw, she fixed it.

After another relatively fast recovery period, I had a properly functioning ICD and felt well again. I was grateful for the quick repair and expertise that had made it possible.

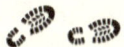

STEP TO REDUCE ANXIETY AND INCREASE HEART HOPE:

Find ways to serve. By helping others, you'll find unexpected joy and renewed purpose.

CHAPTER 18
Building a Heart-Driven Movement

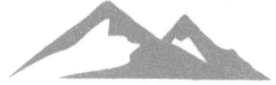

In the early days of Starting Hearts, I had no guidebook or map. The nonprofit world felt like uncharted territory, and every decision came with a sense of uncertainty. I turned to the only constant I knew: daily walks in nature, where I sought guidance from the ground beneath me and Lord above. Those walks became my compass, a quiet assurance that I was being led, even when the path ahead was unclear.

Back home, I poured every ounce of energy into the cause. I created a website, secured my CPR instructor certification, and invested in top-tier training equipment; the kind used in professional medical programs. The Prestan manikins had built-in feedback monitors to help students master their technique. These tools weren't just practical; they made our classes innovative. Starting Hearts was officially incorporated as a nonprofit, and I opened a bank account and obtained a small business credit card.

I needed a venue for our first training. I remembered the community room at the Eagle County Paramedics office and made the ask. When my shipment of manikins was delayed, paramedics lent me the necessary gear so the class could proceed. That kind of generosity became a recurring theme in small, crucial acts that kept us going.

The flyer I'd posted around town read "Free CPR Training." Normally a $50 value, the word "free" drew five participants to that first class. I stood before them, nervous but steady, and shared my story. Then, I walked them through the AHA HeartSaver CPR/AED course. They listened, asked questions, and offered encouragement. Their enthusiasm and gratitude flamed my passion.

After class, I wrote thank-you notes by hand, included donation receipts for those who gave $10 or $20, and celebrated every small gift as if it were a windfall. I wasn't in this for money. I was in it for the moments that could save lives.

People asked why I didn't charge like other instructors. But for me, it wasn't about profit. It was about purpose. I wanted every person, regardless of income or position, to have access to this training. Life-saving skills shouldn't be a privilege.

I carried a CPR manikin with me everywhere—meetings, expos, coffee shops—its plastic head poking out of my tote like a curious companion. People couldn't help but notice and ask questions, so I'd share my story. Sometimes, they'd try a few compressions on the spot. Other times, they just listened, wide-eyed and inspired. These spontaneous conversations planted seeds of awareness across the community.

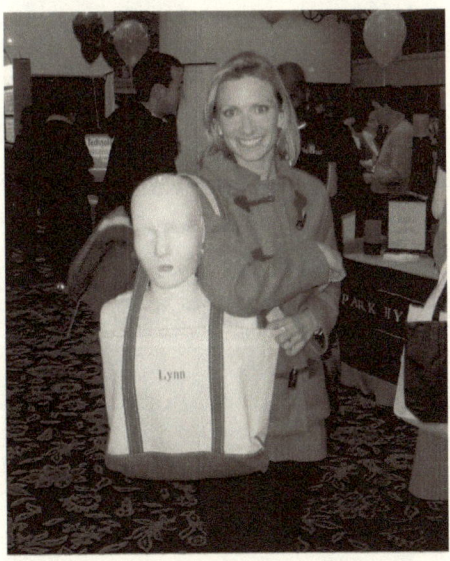

The early days of Starting Hearts.

I joined the Vail Valley Partnership, volunteered at local events, and served on the boards of several nonprofit organizations. I joined Toastmasters to sharpen my presentation skills. One of my most grounding roles was at Vail Health Hospital, where I delivered cookies to patients. In those brief exchanges, through a smile, a soft word, or a silent presence, I connected with the hurting.

Eventually, I joined the planning committee for Rural Philanthropy Days, a statewide initiative connecting nonprofits with funders. I helped organize events and gained knowledge in grant writing, governance, and strategic planning. That involvement gave Starting Hearts its first credibility among other organizations.

Then, something extraordinary happened. The AHA took notice. They named me one of their CPR Spokespeople of the Year, alongside my high-profile responder, Ryan Sutter, and his wife, Trista. We did a professional photo shoot, and I shared with them my dream: a mobile CPR classroom that could bring training to people where they were.

That vision became real when I asked the Town of Vail for one of their decommissioned buses. To my surprise, they donated the vehicle outright. It was a bold move, but the right one.

Matt and I checked out the bus and envisioned it as the HeartRod, a mobile training unit. I studied for and passed the necessary commercial driver's license test. Then scheduled a physical with my doctor.

She was ready to sign off—until she hit the final page, outlining a defibrillator clause. Pacemakers were allowed. ICDs were not. And mine was both.

I blinked back tears. My vision—my calling—hung in the balance.

She was kind, but firm. "It's all over your records. If I sign this, I could lose my license."

Then she offered a workaround: find a doctor at another practice who didn't know my history.

It felt wrong. And it was. Providing false information on the application was a criminal offense that could result in jail time and fines. But I was desperate.

I reasoned that the rule was about passenger safety. My intent was to drive the bus from point A to B and park it. I wasn't transporting anyone. Though my intent was never to break the law, I was caught between rules designed for passenger safety and a mission I believed could save lives.

So, the appointment was made. Without mentioning the small defibrillator detail, I got the signature.

It's not something I'm proud of. But sometimes, the instructed path gets deep, keeping you from the destination. And I was committed to finding another way.

And it was worth it!

The HeartRod became a moving billboard in our community. We gutted the interior, raised the floors, added curtains, rewired the AV system, and hung a disco ball from the ceiling. A friend helped paint the outside with flames, hearts, and wings. We even had beanbag chairs inside for sitting. Over the rear door, I placed a pewter cross—one that didn't really look like a cross—and prayed for every life that would enter.

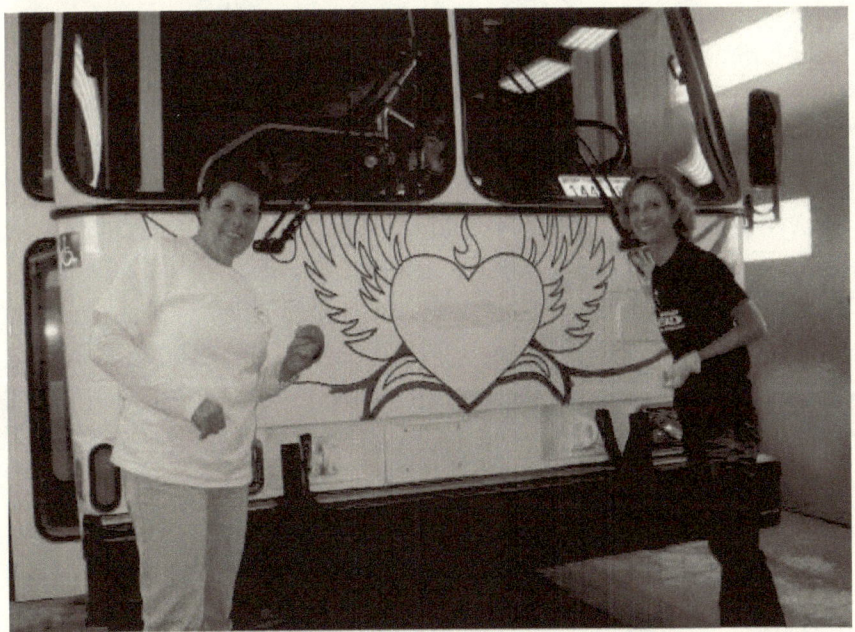

Natalie Zuckerman helping me paint the HeartRod.

The HeartRod wasn't just functional. It was joyful. It sparked curiosity and spread our message through parades, training sessions, and community events. Kids called it "the bumpin' bus," and a student coined our unofficial motto: "If it's bumpin', we're pumpin'!"

Yet, our CPR training had to evolve to stay effective and engaging. Students needed real-world circumstances. So, we customized scenarios: at the dinner table, skiing on the mountain, or in bed. We dressed manikins in casual clothing and gave them names like Joey the skier, who wore no helmet, and Suzy Q, the sunbather with balloons in her bikini, making the training more relatable. We also added Big Fred, a manikin that required more strength for compressions, and CasPeR, our CPR dog. Incorporating clothing and different body types brought a new level of consideration and realism.

I also shared a real-life example of an elderly couple from my church. The wife, dependent on oxygen and with limited mobility, had to use her foot to perform chest compressions when her husband went into cardiac arrest. It was an unconventional response, but a powerful reminder that in critical moments, people must improvise. The audience appreciated the insight because it reflected reality. Very few cardiac arrests unfold like the textbook scenarios practiced in training. Real-life responses are unpredictable and require quick thinking under pressure.

We also developed a new mantra. Inspired by 'Stop, Drop, and Roll,' I crafted a new, memorable message to guide the public: CALL. PUSH. SHOCK. It was direct, empowering, and easy to remember.

With help from Graham, the lead paramedic from my cardiac arrest, we built a short curriculum around it. People were amazed that saving a life didn't require medical training, just a willingness to act.

However, defibrillator access remained a major challenge—not because of the technology, but fear and misunderstanding. We had to work hard to undo the misconceptions the public had developed over decades. When defibrillators first became available to civilians, they were intimidating, misrepresented, and underutilized. Many bystanders hesitated, worried they might shock someone unnecessarily or be held liable. They didn't realize an AED only delivers a shock for deadly rhythms like ventricular fibrillation, and all 50 states have Good Samaritan laws protecting responders. Ironically, lawsuits have occurred *because* a defibrillator wasn't used.

At the time, there weren't even cabinets designed to store AEDs outside. So, we created our own. Our first unit was assembled with electrical components sourced by Chief McGee, who, in his role as deputy fire chief and inspector, knew practically every building owner in town. With a quick conversation and a twirl of his gray handlebar mustache, he could usually convince anyone to install them. We encouraged people to move devices out from behind locked doors and into public view—mounted on light posts for quick, visible access within a lifesaving four-minute window.

At some point, I stopped using the acronym "AED" unless I was communicating with someone in the industry and started calling them what they are: defibrillators. Or simply, a "defib." The word fib—short for fibrillation—is rooted in many languages, and that shared linguistic thread made it more universally understood. Frankly, the term AED has always bothered me. It's vague, easily confused with other acronyms, and does it really matter to the layperson that it's automated or external? What matters is that it restarts a heart. That's the core truth.

We also learned about PulsePoint, a reverse 911 app that notifies CPR-trained citizens about nearby cardiac arrests and maps defibrillators. I worked with public safety agencies and dispatch, laying the groundwork for future integration. I also created a registry of trained responders I called "Neighbor Savers."

Starting Hearts was no longer just an idea. It was becoming a movement.

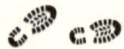

STEP TO REDUCE ANXIETY AND INCREASE HEART HOPE:

Do things differently. What once worked may no longer be the solution.

CHAPTER 19
No Data, No Dollars

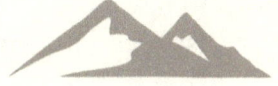

Despite the growing impact, not everything came easily. Convincing donors and foundations to support us required more than passion. It required proof. Without measurable outcomes, our story, however moving, was not enough. I was repeatedly told we needed data.

As I poured my energy into Starting Hearts, doubt seeped in. Regardless of my conviction, the nonprofit wasn't reaching the goals I had envisioned. I wondered if all the effort and resources were worth it.

Kelly, a respected paramedic with her own story of survival, encouraged me to look at Seattle's Medic One system. Internationally recognized for its exceptional cardiac arrest outcomes, King County, WA, consistently achieves survival rates nearly double the national average.

She recommended *Resuscitate!* by Dr. Mickey Eisenberg, which outlines the science and strategy of saving lives through a coordinated, high-performing approach. One core principle stood out: what gets measured gets improved.

And the most critical component of all: systematic data collection and analysis. By gathering details from cardiac arrest incidents, stakeholders can identify trends, response times, survival rates, and measure impact.

The importance of data struck me deeply. As I explored the issue, I found a lack of comprehensive reporting at the national level. The Centers for Disease Control (CDC) did not classify cardiac arrest as a notifiable disease, meaning agencies are not required to report it as a cause of death. This exclusion results in mass vacancies of data, hindering an understanding of the epidemic, which leads to inadequate prevention measures.

That led to CARES—Cardiac Arrest Registry to Enhance Survival. In partnership with Eagle County Paramedic Services, Starting Hearts funded our community's participation. The reporting system gave us something we hadn't had before: data and a way to quantify prevalence.

Through a local survey, we uncovered critical knowledge gaps. Most residents couldn't distinguish between cardiac arrest and a heart attack. Even fewer knew how to locate or use a defibrillator.

The findings confirmed what we had long suspected: the public was unprepared to respond. Now, we had both the evidence, and the responsibility, to change that.

To move from inspiration to sustainability, I needed more structure. I joined the Vail Leadership Institute's Leaders Lab, a transformative opportunity that helped me build Starting Hearts into a strategic, scalable organization. Twice a week, I sat alongside other entrepreneurs in the for-profit world and absorbed lessons on finance, leadership, and messaging. During a reflective assignment, we were asked to write our epitaphs. Mine read: "Lynn saved earthly and eternal lives." That line became my North Star—a quiet promise I returned to in moments of doubt.

The mentorship I received helped me refine our mission, develop a formal business plan, and articulate our goals clearly and concisely. It paid off sooner than expected.

One CPR session included a young woman named Jade. Afterward, her mom, Andie, proposed organizing a community fundraiser. We began planning "All You Need is Heart," an ambitious Valentine's Day event featuring Dr. Terry Gordon, the AHA's National Physician of the Year. What began as an idea quickly evolved into a full-scale campaign featuring heart health screenings, CPR demonstrations, a Beatles tribute band, and the symbolic launch of our AED Adoption Auction.

In preparing for the event, we met regularly to pin hundreds of existing and proposed defibrillator locations on community maps, organize volunteers, and spread the word. During the planning, I connected with three powerhouse couples who considered our community their second home—and who would play pivotal roles in our success.

The Mowers, Morton and Toby, brought both credibility and compassion. Morton, the renowned cardiologist and the co-inventor of the implantable defibrillator, who graciously agreed to speak at the event, and Toby, a dedicated philanthropist energized support. The Mowers' presence alone served as a powerful validation of our mission, and his endorsement opened doors we never imagined.

The Tobins came with deep roots in the ICD industry. Cathy was a former cardiac nurse, and Jim was the retired CEO of Boston Scientific, the device implanted in my chest.

The Markowitzes—Alan was a skilled cardiac surgeon, and Cathy was an experienced nurse and nonprofit leader.

All three couples became committed champions—funding marketing campaigns, lending their names to our cause, taking part in committees, and standing beside us as we expanded our reach.

Though we only saw three AEDs adopted that morning, the event did something bigger: it established public awareness. People no longer needed convincing. They leaned forward, asked thoughtful questions, and offered to help. We gained credibility and built lasting momentum, along with connections that would bring on the next chapter.

That momentum carried into the planning of our second annual event. Our goal was clear: raise $25,000 to integrate PulsePoint technology to officially launch Neighbor Saver. These programs were our next evolution, tying together training, access, and available responders. PulsePoint would formalize our community database and notify trained citizens nearby of cardiac arrests in real-time.

Carolyn—whose niece tragically died from cardiac arrest just after marrying at twenty-seven, a haunting mirror of my occurrence—joined me on a local radio show to share our vision. After the broadcast, Carolyn's longtime friend Drew reached out. He asked all the right questions: "What's your budget? How do you sustain this? Are you collaborating with other agencies? What's your business plan?"

Thanks to Leaders Lab, I had the answers. I explained the implementation fee, ongoing maintenance costs, and our plan to secure sponsors. Drew was impressed. He committed to funding PulsePoint and adopting two AEDs on the spot. That single conversation transformed our capacity to act.

The connection reminded me that success comes from an equal balance of making things happen and letting things happen. The next big break could come from anywhere—and it often did when I least expected it.

We formalized our board of directors by bringing together those who had supported us from the start. Jacquie contributed countless volunteer hours; Carolyn, a deep personal loss; Christine offered ties to Vail Health; Russell, business expertise; and Ilene, insight from Vail Resorts. We also welcomed the first responders who saved my life—Sue, Capt. Spell, and Graham. Their collective experience helped shape our strategic direction and credibility when we needed it most.

We also took critical legal steps to secure trademarks for our signature programs: CALL. PUSH. SHOCK., Nearest AED, and Neighbor Saver. These weren't just brand elements. They were the foundation of our identity and the message we conveyed.

Amid all this progress, one constant anchored me: gratitude. I filled drawers with notecards and pens. Whether someone gave $5 or donated a venue, they received a handwritten thank-you. The cards featured a watercolor of diverse people forming a heart, a visual expression that cardiac arrest impacts everyone.

Gratitude changed my outlook, and often, my outcomes. It reminded me that every meeting, every donation, and every setback had a purpose. The actual gift wasn't the recognition or funding. It was the people who walked alongside me. Their belief in our mission turned my private pain into a public message of hope.

Starting Hearts began as a personal calling to redeem what I had survived. But as it grew, it evolved into something much larger—a movement powered by conviction, compassion, and collaboration. Every conversation, class, and campaign brought us closer to the vision we held: a community where no one dies from preventable cardiac arrest because someone nearby was ready to act.

Experiencing both the highs and lows taught me: rejection is inevitable. People often fear what they don't understand, and some even renounce it. But when you encounter those who won't accept you or your message, don't let that stop you. Instead, let it propel you toward the ones who are ready to hear it—because they're the ones who truly need it.

What once felt like a mess had become a mission others could rally around. The work had matured into an operation. We had data, direction, and a team behind us. We were stepping up and stepping in—proof that ordinary people can do extraordinary things when they refuse to give up.

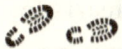

STEP TO REDUCE ANXIETY AND INCREASE HEART HOPE:

Build structure. Success happens through small, consistent actions and the support of others.

CHAPTER 20
Signs From Above

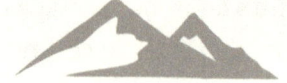

It was one of those fog-drenched hikes through the aspen grove, where the trail seemed to vanish beneath my feet. I had walked for hours, only to find myself in unfamiliar territory, with no clear path forward. Frustration bubbled as I stared at the dense vegetation around me, each tree and branch blending into the next. I felt disoriented, unsure of how far I should keep going.

That moment in the woods paralleled my position in life. Even after several years, my commitment to Starting Hearts was still entirely voluntary. While Matt worked tirelessly to keep us financially afloat in an area with a high cost of living and extreme recreational activities, I poured everything I had into building the organization. Living on one income was challenging, yet we always scraped by.

By early 2014, Starting Hearts had grown enough that I could begin drawing a modest payment—$1,000 per month—for what often felt like sixty-hour workweeks. Even as the nonprofit gained momentum, I couldn't ignore a growing ache. While other women in my circle were stepping into motherhood, I wrestled with feelings of inadequacy and longing.

I straddled the line between celebrating the beauty in others' blessings and quietly mourning what I had yet to receive. Their good news stirred a bittersweet pang, a tender reminder of what hadn't come my way. In those moments, I had to redirect my perspective: someone else's success didn't mean my failure. I was walking a different path, one defined by purpose—and by saving lives. *What could be more meaningful than that?* I reminded myself.

Throughout, there were still moments of joy—skiing, friendships, cribbage games, and the unconditional love of our spaniels, Sadie and Charlie. Matt and I had grown closer, leaning on each other in the face of disappointments and uncertainty.

Putting motherhood on hold and stepping away from my career for the past five years to build Starting Hearts tested both my patience and perseverance. Life, I was learning, is a continuous cycle of waiting and learning. Embracing that process didn't come quickly.

Though Starting Hearts thrived with community support and increasing funds, I felt restless. I needed direction—a sign—and then I noticed one.

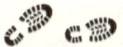

I ran into Dr. Skaggs—the obstetrician who had cared for me during our first loss—repeatedly around town: at the post office, the grocery store, even walking through the neighborhood. Her presence stirred something in me. She had moved away for a while, so seeing her again felt like more than a coincidence. It felt like a quiet charge from above.

I felt the pull of possibility each time I passed new mothers pushing strollers. I imagined my round belly, the miracle of life growing within me. With cautious hope, I made an appointment with Dr. Skaggs.

She was warm and reassuring. She believed it was still possible for us to conceive, despite my being 34, and referred us to a high-risk specialist in Summit County.

Dr. Gutierrez welcomed us with gentle confidence. A native of Mexico who spent half of his time caring for underserved communities in Mexico City. His service and kindness gave us peace of mind.

After confirming that everything looked optimal, he prescribed a fertility injection, and we entered the next chapter of our journey. Matt gave me the shot himself. Then came the waiting—a long, anxious time when hope and uncertainty danced together.

Finally, the day arrived: I missed my period.

With hearts pounding, we scheduled a follow-up appointment. Dr. Gutierrez didn't keep us in suspense. "You're pregnant!" he beamed. It was too early to hear a heartbeat, but the joy was instant and overwhelming. Another appointment was scheduled for two weeks later. Haunted by our first loss . . . Matt insisted on being at every visit.

On the now-familiar thirty-minute drive, we allowed ourselves to feel hopeful.

Dr. Gutierrez entered the room with his characteristic warmth— lighthearted but never dismissive. He glanced at the monitor and smiled gently before asking, "Do you want the good or bad news first?"

"Uh . . . I guess the bad news," I said hesitantly.

"You're pregnant with twins!" he announced.

My jaw dropped. "That's the bad news?"

He grinned. "The good news? You're pregnant!"

It was surreal—exhilarating, humbling, and laced with awe. He explained that the road ahead wouldn't be easy. A twin pregnancy came with more complications and responsibility. But to me, it was perfect—one pregnancy, two children. The timing, the meaning—it all felt like a righteous reward for our patience.

I dove headfirst into research on twin pregnancy—reading everything from double strollers to nursery configurations. But I reminded myself not to get ahead. We were only eight weeks in. First, we had to get my electrophysiologist, Dr. Prager, involved.

Dr. Prager could detect heartbeats at our next visit with just a stethoscope. It was astonishing. We rushed to Walgreens to buy the only dusty stethoscope on the shelf so I could listen at home. But without training, all I heard was silence.

Still, hope pulsed through every cell of my body. I prayed daily, thanking God for the pregnancy, yet pleading for protection. The fear of another loss hovered close.

We returned for another appointment a few weeks later, and I sensed unease in the room.

Dr. Gutierrez gently shared the news: one twin had stopped growing, its heartbeat no longer detectable. The surviving baby, however, was healthy and developing well.

The familiar sting of loss returned. Questions swirled in our minds—would this affect the other baby? Was another heartbreak on the horizon?

Dr. Gutierrez reassured us. This type of loss wasn't uncommon. The body would naturally absorb the tissue, allowing the remaining baby to grow. We mourned the dream of twins, but focused on nurturing the life we still carried.

Determined to ease my anxiety, I purchased a fetal Doppler monitor for home use. Each day, I searched for the rhythm that would bring reassurance. Slowly, the surviving baby's heartbeat grew stronger, and so did our hope.

At twelve weeks, confidence took root. We started telling close family and friends. Dr. Gutierrez, recognizing the complexity of my case, referred me to an even higher-risk obstetrician at the University of Colorado in Denver. The urban environment, with its industrial air and sprawling medical campuses nestled at the foot of the Rockies, felt both distant and vital. Dr. Jones was calm, competent, and deeply reassuring. Her team would oversee the delivery, prepared for every potential complication. After reviewing my condition, she offered words that stayed with me: "If, for some unlikely reason, your device was to fire, the baby would likely survive."

She even gave me her cell phone number in case of an emergency. Dr. Jones's confidence and accessibility were supportive.

As news of our pregnancy spread and my belly began to show, we drove down the familiar winding highway to Denver for my cousin

Arthur's baby shower. As we descended from the mountains, the city emerged—clouds rising above the skyline in the morning sun, shimmering with mystery and promise. It was a chance to celebrate motherhood alongside others at last, to feel part of a joy I had long yearned for.

But on that routine stretch of I-70, something changed.

I was typing on my laptop when a sudden hammering force slammed into my chest, firing every nerve in an instant. As quickly as it happened, it was over. I looked up to process the unsettling interruption.

"Are we in an accident?" I gasped; eyes were wide.

Matt glanced over, alarmed. "No, Lynn, are you okay?"

Although shaken, I knew I had to explain calmly and carefully. "I think my defibrillator just went off."

Confused and concerned, he asked for details. "Are you sure?"

"I don't know. It felt like a giant kick to my chest," I said. "I'm okay, but we need to call 911."

I dialed with trembling hands. The dispatcher instructed us to exit the highway immediately—an ambulance was en route. We pulled off at Exit 253, Chief Hosa.

As we waited, fear consumed me. What was happening to my heart? Was our baby in danger? Was I dying?

The ambulance arrived quickly. As the paramedics lifted me onto the gurney, my ICD shocked me again. The pain was sharp and instant. I cried out—not from the sensation itself, but from the fear, the isolation, losing control. The doors closed.

Matt's face was foreboding, pressed against the glass of the ambulance window. Tears streamed down his face. He was watching his wife and baby disappear into the unknown. We both feared the worst.

They connected a twelve-lead EKG inside the ambulance and monitored my vital signs. My heart rhythm looked stable, beating at 65 bpm. Still, they warned, the device might shock me again if it was misreading signals.

I begged them to stop it, but it was out of their control until we reached the hospital.

Once there, a team was waiting. The emergency doctor quickly applied a large donut-shaped medical magnet over the device, deactivating its shocking function. I hadn't known that was possible, but now I understood why ICD patients are warned to avoid magnets.

Relief washed over me as I realized I was safe—my heart was calm, and, hopefully, the baby was still okay.

Diagnosing the issue took time. Admitted on a Saturday, Matt and I spent the weekend in a haze of uncertainty, praying for answers.

Finally, the problem was discovered on Monday: a fractured defibrillator lead. The break in the ventricular wire had caused the device to misread electrical "noise" as a dangerous rhythm, delivering unnecessary shocks.

During an ultrasound to check on our baby, Matt and I held our breath. To our great relief, he appeared unaffected.

But the path forward was far from simple.

Repairing the lead would require surgery, which is too challenging for a pregnant woman. Instead, the team recommended deactivating the defibrillating function while maintaining the pacing feature. It wasn't ideal, but it was the safest option.

To compensate, I was prescribed a wearable defibrillator—the Zoll LifeVest. The idea of wearing it was incomprehensible, especially while pregnant. Designed to detect cardiac arrest and deliver lifesaving shocks, it was bulky, uncomfortable, and overwhelming.

The vest fastened just below my chest and above my growing belly with wide Velcro straps. Suspenders crossed over my shoulders, securing six electrodes that continuously read my heart rhythm, all connected by wires to a five-pound battery pack and monitor. Two large pads, one on my chest and one on my back, were ready to deliver a shock at any time. If the system detected a dangerous rhythm, it would vibrate, sound an alarm, and give me thirty seconds to simultaneously press two buttons to disarm it.

I hated it.

But Matt and Dr. Prager insisted I wear it.

Wearing the LifeVest meant constant maintenance. Matt, my faithful partner in everything, cleaned the electrodes each night with Q-tips and alcohol, then applied just enough lotion to keep them from drying out. Too little or too much moisture or buildup prompted false readings.

Even with his meticulous efforts, the vest seemed to have its own mind. It would vibrate and sound its sirens several times a day, threatening an impending intervention. Each time, my heart pounded as I scrambled to press the buttons to avoid being shocked.

Pregnancy was already complicated. The LifeVest made it so much more challenging. Sleeping was nearly impossible. As soon as I drifted off, the vest would go off again.

The physical discomfort and itching were persistent, and the emotional toll wore me down. I lived in a constant state of hyper-vigilance. Even moments of peace were clouded by the anticipation of the next alarm.

One day, my dad showed up with a small gift that brought unexpected comfort: the back scratcher I had given him as a child for Christmas. He had saved it all these years. Now, it soothed the itches beneath the vest—and reminded me of the love and support carrying me through.

Still wearing the LifeVest, I remained immersed in my work with Starting Hearts. I continued teaching CPR classes and preparing for our next big event, Art for Hearts.

This time, we had the honor of showcasing the world's largest private collection of original Rembrandt etchings—curated by the Mowers. With over 80 works, it offered a rare glimpse into Rembrandt's prolific career as a master printmaker.

The Mowers' generosity overwhelmed me. Art for Hearts elevated the stature of Starting Hearts, aligning our mission with world-class culture and cause.

But as the event approached, another scare arrived.

One morning, there was blood in my discharge.

Panic surged through me. Matt was out on a bike ride, so I called my mom, sobbing.

"Mom! I'm bleeding—I can't lose this baby!"

She stayed calm and prayed with me over the phone.

When Matt returned, heart pounding, he told me what he had seen on his ride: a mother deer, a father, and a baby crossing the trail before him. It was a quiet sign. We took comfort in it.

Dr. Gutierrez confirmed the bleeding was minor—nothing to worry about. Still, the emotional whiplash of parenthood had begun long before birth.

My pregnancy progressed, and the need to increase the size of the LifeVest became unavoidable. Overwhelmed by the discomfort, anxiety, and anticipation of the procedure, I arrived at Dr. Prager's office in tears.

Seeing my distress, the technician offered kind reassurance. "This is just a minor blip on the screen of your life. Trust me—once that baby is born, you won't even remember this happened."

Her words didn't erase the frustration and fear, but they gave me perspective. I was nearing the final stretch of this long, demanding period. I knew I had to find the strength to push through. Our child would need a resilient mother, so that became my focus.

Other than the persistent alarms and frustrations with the LifeVest, the rest of my pregnancy unfolded without significant complications. I was fortunate to be spared the typical discomforts and ailments. I felt well. And I felt loved.

The Cracked Pots ladies—who had once surrounded me in my longing—were now surrounding me in celebration. They had prayed for me during the hard seasons, watched me surrender my life and purpose, and now they were lifting me through this sacred period.

As summer neared its end, they surprised me with a baby shower, an act of love that included a generous collection for us to use however we needed.

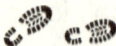

Sometimes, we find ourselves in need of direction, unsure of what's next. We push forward mindlessly, believing we can muscle through on our own. But what often feels like coincidence is divine alignment—a subtle nudge, an unexpected encounter, or a quiet whisper in our hearts reminding us we're not lost after all.

Those signs—however they appear—are gentle affirmations that we're still on the right path, even if the way forward isn't clear. They remind us to stay open, trust, and keep walking, one step at a time.

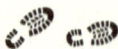

STEP TO REDUCE ANXIETY AND INCREASE HEART HOPE:

Coincidences are signs. Notice and follow the quiet directions.

CHAPTER 21
Lightening the Load

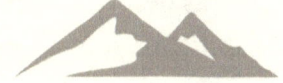

The higher I climbed, the heavier my pack felt. What began as a carefully planned load now felt like a burden dragging me backward. Each commitment to Starting Hearts was no longer just a task—it became a daily strain, both emotionally and physically, that slowly wore me down.

The trail grew steeper. The air thinned. My steps slowed. I stopped more often—not just to catch my breath, but to ask myself an honest question: *Could I keep climbing if I didn't let something go?*

Starting Hearts had reached a turning point. With financial support in place—funding my modest monthly payment and a growing team—the organization was positioned for growth. But as my due date neared, I knew it was time to focus fully on becoming a mother—and to pass the torch. Starting Hearts needed someone who could lead it forward.

I placed a classified ad for an executive director.

Applications came in. With guidance from Sue and Capt. Spell, whom I now call Jim, we started the interview process. One name kept rising to the top: Alan Himelfarb.

A contact at the *Vail Daily* had recommended him. Alan intrigued me—not just for his impressive resume, including work with Lee Iacocca, but also because he was married to the woman who had inspired me at the Breast Cancer Awareness Luncheon years before. He invited me to lunch at a local bistro.

When I walked in, the LifeVest strapped across my body, I immediately sensed a connection. Alan sat ready with a folder full of ideas. As we talked, I learned his father had died from cardiac arrest at the kitchen table when Alan was a child. That memory had never left him, and it fueled his desire to help.

He wanted to use his skills for something that mattered. And everything he said aligned with our mission.

We continued with formal interviews and board protocols, but Alan was the one.

His energy, strategic thinking, and personal connection to our cause made him the right leader. When he accepted the position, it felt like confirmation from above—a sign that this wasn't just a hire, but a continuation of the mission.

With only weeks before the baby's arrival, I poured everything I knew into Alan—CPR training, AED access, funding structures, and partnerships. He absorbed it all, and when the Third Annual *All You Need is Heart* event came around, Alan stepped in and led confidently.

He brought extra energy, fresh credibility, and a bold vision. Starting Hearts was in capable hands. The torch had been passed, and I could finally breathe—and release what I'd carried for so long.

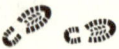

With the leadership transition complete, my focus turned fully toward the next chapter: motherhood.

We planned to name our son Thomas Froeschle Blake.

Thomas was a family name on both sides—my father, grandfather, Matt's grandfather, and uncle all shared it. It also carried a spiritual connection, honoring the disciple who doubted and then believed.

His middle name, Froeschle, was chosen for Sue, who saved my life and made this moment possible. It means "little frog" in German, and soon, a frog theme found its way into the nursery. Though Sue never had children of her own, her legacy would live on in our family forever.

In November, Margaret, and my friends Adrienne, Chelsey, and Rachel hosted another baby shower—a beautiful celebration overflowing with car seats, strollers, blankets, and clothes.

We were surrounded by love and support, laughter echoing through the room. But beneath the surface joy, a quiet unease lingered—reminders of what we'd been through and what still lay ahead.

Chelsey, radiant and smiling, had just given birth to her second child four months earlier. But something in her seemed . . . off. She was thinner than I'd ever seen her. Ben and the kids hadn't come with her. And beneath her glowing exterior was a quiet sadness I couldn't name—at least not yet.

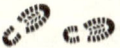

STEP TO REDUCE ANXIETY AND INCREASE HEART HOPE:

Ask for help. Life isn't meant to be done alone; people want to support you.

CHAPTER 22
The Final Stretch

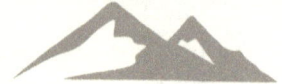

A jagged peak pierced the sky, close enough that it felt like I could reach out and touch it. But as I stood there, legs trembling from the unrelenting climb, I felt the weight of every step it had taken to get here. The summit should have filled me with excitement, yet all I could feel was the burden of the final ascent.

January 2015 marked the arrival of Thomas Froeschle Blake, planned precisely one week before his due date. I would give birth on Friday, have two days to bond and recover, then undergo surgery on Monday to extract and insert new leads and an ICD. The thought of shedding the LifeVest brought immense relief. While my mom suggested keeping it as a memento of the ordeal, I was eager to discard it, ready to leave it behind.

Instead of the LifeVest, the medical team placed traditional defibrillator pads as a precaution in case of cardiac complications during childbirth. Every detail of the delivery had been mapped out to address potential risks.

As the nurses prepared to induce labor, Matt held my hand, our nerves and anticipation quietly swelling.

"Ready to be parents?" the nurse asked, reading our cautious smiles.

Matt's reassuring squeeze offered comfort. The night before, we had soaked in our last hours as a family of two, savoring a shared glass of champagne and lobster cocktail at Elway's in downtown Denver.

Beneath the twinkling lights of Larimer Square, we reflected on our journey and braced for what lay ahead.

Surprisingly, we slept well in our Ritz-Carlton suite—a gift from Matt's work. His persistence and success in real estate had turned our finances around, affording us a few well-earned luxuries.

That night eased our worries and let us acknowledge how far we'd come. I returned Matt's squeeze, ready for what lay before us. It felt like the ultimate resting point before the summit—a pause to gather strength for the last push.

Labor progressed quickly, eased by the epidural. As the seven-hour labor neared its end, a flicker of unease surfaced when the nurses noticed irregularities in the baby's heartbeat.

"Hmmm, it seems there might be some trouble with the baby's heart," one nurse said, her voice tinged with concern.

We watched and waited; the tension mounting. At 1:52 a.m., Thomas emerged, his tiny head blue from the umbilical cord wrapped tightly around his neck. The medical team sprang into action, using forceps to assist the delivery. The intervention caused a perineal tear, a common but painful complication of childbirth.

"We suspect the umbilical cord may have been causing the cardiovascular abnormalities," the doctor explained. "However, given your history and to err on the side of caution, we'll order an EKG in the morning." Her words offered a mix of optimism and warning.

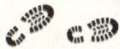

Finally, our dreams had come true. We were blessed with another little miracle—a five-pound, fourteen-ounce bundle of joy. Looking into his inquisitive eyes and holding him for those first few minutes filled me with awe. But all too soon, the nurses whisked him away for routine exams and cleaning.

As they stitched up the tear and removed the epidural, I stood to use the restroom, and a sharp headache consumed me. Moments later, the room spun, and I felt consciousness slipping away. The nurses rushed in, catching me before I collapsed, cracking an ammonia inhalant beneath my nose to jolt me awake. Weak and disoriented, I was guided to the toilet, trying to steady myself.

The doctor recommended a blood transfusion because of significant blood loss, but I resisted, unsettled by the idea of foreign blood. Meanwhile, Matt cradled Thomas, a steady presence amid the hysterics. Well into the "golden hour," when I finally felt strong enough, Thomas was returned to my arms, but the throbbing in my head was so intense, I struggled to savor the moment fully.

Undeterred by it being the middle of the night, my parents, Olgie and Grumps, rushed to the hospital to meet their grandchild. Their presence brought joy, but the vicious headache refused to let up. Nevertheless, we all tried to rest, though for me, sleep was elusive.

By daylight, the pain remained relentless. Nurses administered medication, and while it took the edge off, it wasn't enough to let me enjoy the newborn bonding, skin-to-skin, I had long imagined. As Thomas underwent his heart assessment, I watched the nurses place twelve electrodes across his infant frame, covering nearly every inch of his tiny, fragile body. The image was hauntingly familiar—a miniature echo of the tests I'd undergone myself. My heart ached, hoping he would be spared the cardiovascular battles that had defined so much of my past.

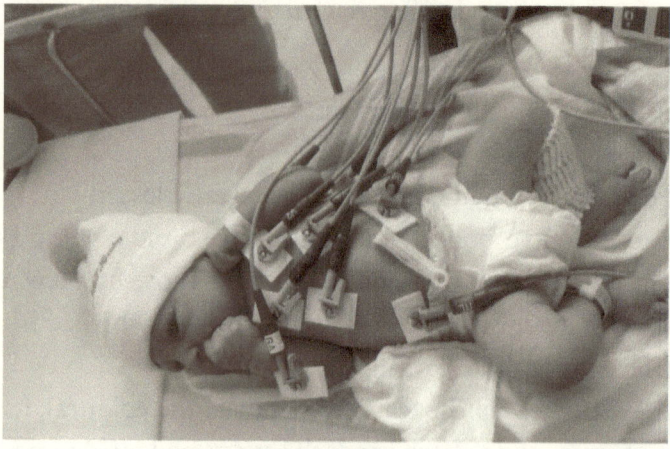

Thomas receiving his first EKG.

The results were reassuring: aside from a small murmur—common in newborns—his heart appeared healthy.

Just as I tried to relax, a knock at the door startled me. To my surprise, my in-laws, Joanne and David, had flown in, excited to meet Thomas and support Matt during my surgery. While their presence was well-meaning and usually welcome, I was in so much pain that all I wanted was quiet, just Matt, Thomas, and me.

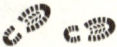

The stimulation became too much. Even having my mother and mother-in-law nearby couldn't soothe the pounding in my head. A concerned nurse floated a rare diagnosis: pneumocephalus—an air bubble in the spine, potentially left by the epidural.

Of course, I thought—another uncommon complication for my already rare medical file.

The suggested remedy was a blood patch, a procedure where my blood would be drawn and re-injected into my spine to close the air pocket. There were no guarantees it would work. I was beyond frustrated—tears flowed freely as I grappled with the prospect of yet another needle, another procedure.

But the headache robbed me of the most precious moments—my first days with Thomas. Desperate for relief, I agreed. With Matt by my side, I braced for a second epidural.

This time, the relief was immediate. After thirty-six hours of blinding pain, I could finally breathe, rest, and begin bonding with our baby—if only for a little while.

The second phase of our high-risk birthing plan involved an intricate cardiovascular lead extraction to replace my fractured ICD wires. Because there was no space left in my arteries, the existing atrial and ventricular leads had to be entirely removed—a daunting procedure that was still relatively new and carried a 5 percent mortality rate.

The gravity of that statistic sank in heavily. I had just given birth.

I was still weak, still sore. And now I was facing a surgery that would stop and restart my heart—a reality that some patients didn't survive.

Part of me wanted to halt everything right there. I considered postponing the operation and living with the LifeVest for a few more months. I craved a break—just a few weeks to catch my breath and enjoy our son. The thought of one more step, let alone the final push to the summit, felt impossible. My body was screaming for rest.

Matt and I talked late into the night, weighing our options, looking for clarity. What if I died on the operating table? Would Matt be left to raise Thomas alone? The thought of missing everything I had fought so hard to live for was dreadful to consider.

But we had come too far. We couldn't stop now. I needed something to shift the fear.

I called my parents. My mother, steady and strong, encouraged me to read Psalm 118.

Matt and I opened the Bible app and read aloud. Then, verse 17 leaped off the screen and into my soul: *"I will not die but live, and will proclaim what the Lord has done."*

Peace washed over me. My fear didn't vanish completely, but the panic receded. I knew, somehow, that I would live—and that it was time to keep climbing.

The next morning, I lay on the gurney in the surgical prep area, grasping my loved ones tightly, knowing these could be our last moments together before the anesthesia carried me into the unknown. With tearful hugs and kisses, I said goodbye to Matt—Thomas swaddled in his arms—and to our parents.

As the surgery began, time stretched endlessly for my family.

The procedure was delicate and complex. Surgeons inserted catheters into both femoral arteries, threading tiny lasers up through to my heart to remove the scar tissue surrounding the damaged leads. Once the tissue was cleared, the old leads were freed and disconnected.

New leads were then inserted through the veins and connected to a fresh ICD generator, which was secured beneath the same skin and muscle. To ensure the new device worked properly, my heart was briefly stopped and restarted—an event I would not remember, but one that everyone else waited through with bated breath.

Meanwhile, in the waiting room, each family member coped in their own way. Conversations came and went. Silent prayers were lifted. The weight of uncertainty hung in the air.

Then Matt's absence was noted.

Concerned, his father looked outside and found him running in the frigid January air. It was his way of processing and staying grounded in the unknown.

Finally, after what felt like an eternity, the news came: the surgery had been a success. I was alive and recovering in the ICU.

When I awoke, gratitude flooded my body. Exhausted and groggy, I still managed a weary smile. I would need time to fully recover, but I had made it.

The next twenty-four hours passed in a blur of monitoring and rest. But even as I recovered, another worry crept in: I hadn't been able to breastfeed Thomas. In those critical first days, that connection was essential. Still under sedation, I couldn't nurse him, so my mother and a compassionate nurse stepped in, pumping milk to engage the supply.

Matt cared for Thomas with tenderness and calm, feeding him with donated breast milk from the hospital. His gentle presence eased my guilt and allowed me to focus on healing.

Though I could barely move, I was allowed brief visits with Thomas in the ICU. Holding him—even for a moment—reminded me why I'd fought so hard. Because of the medications I was taking, he couldn't breastfeed right away. I pumped and dumped, attempting to preserve the rhythm of milk production until I could nourish him.

Eventually, I was transferred back to the maternity floor. There, I continued my recovery while learning how to care for Thomas with one functional arm.

The nurses, deeply moved by our circumstances, nicknamed me "Miracle Mama." I didn't feel like a miracle—but I knew we had survived something extraordinary. Everyone loves a good miracle story. We just prefer to avoid being in a circumstance where we need one, and that was true now.

After a week that felt like a lifetime, the moment had finally arrived—we were leaving the hospital behind, bringing home our much-anticipated baby, Thomas. Matt carefully secured him in his car seat and I settled into the back, our hearts swelling with love and trepidation as we gazed at our newborn son.

The drive ahead triggered a rush of anxiety within me—could I handle the responsibility of this tiny life, especially with my fresh scar and lack of experience? How was I going to care for him and myself when we returned home?

Minutes into the drive, a gush of panic swept over me, propelling me to move to the front seat beside Matt. With each passing mile, the anxiety ebbed, replaced by the peace of our sleeping baby.

Once home, I savored the simple pleasures of showering and settling in, grateful to be in the place and time we longed to be. When my parents arrived with Sadie and Charlie, the introduction scene was heartwarming, if somewhat comical—Sadie's indifference contrasting with Charlie's eager curiosity, while Thomas looked wide-eyed, taking in the foreign furry creatures.

That evening, as we snuggled on the sofa, the burdens of the past nine months seemed to lift, replaced by contentment. Yet, later, as I attempted to climb into bed with Thomas cradled in my arms, a surge of dizziness overtook me, causing us both to tumble to the floor.

In that moment of fear and frustration, water welled up in both of our eyes. My embrace protected Thomas, but he remained frightened by the sudden fall and let out loud cries. I was emotionally distraught, questioning the fairness of all my pain, and could no longer suppress the tears.

Worried, Matt rushed in upon hearing all the commotion. Wiping the drips away, I assured him we were okay. Now safely cradling Thomas in bed, a realization struck me with clarity—setting aside the unconventional challenges, I was blessed beyond measure.

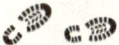

Two weeks into settling into our new routine, Matt's parents, affectionately known as Grammy and Grandpa, arrived to help. Several nights into the serenity of their stay, a haunting cry shattered the peace—a sharp, anguished sound from one dog echoed through the house. Since Sadie and Charlie stayed in their room, we assumed they would tend to it and drifted back to sleep, unaware of the tragedy unfolding.

As I tried to feed Thomas in bed in the early morning, I caught the emotion of Matt's tearful gaze before he spoke. With a sinking heart, I whispered the words I already knew: "Sadie's gone."

Matt lowered his head and confirmed, "Yes."

Time seemed to freeze as the reality sank in.

Though devastated, I was still recovering from surgery and caring for Thomas, so Matt took the lead. With gentle hands and a heavy heart, he wrapped Sadie in the blanket she had slept on and carried her to the vet.

Sadie had been our steady companion for nine years. While the signs of aging had hinted at health troubles, her sudden passing blindsided us. We had imagined many more years with her, but it seemed Sadie had other plans.

One thought eased our grief: Sadie had stayed just long enough to meet Thomas, as if she knew her work was complete. She wasn't just a pet—she was our confidant, our comforter, the one who had carried us to the blessing now nestled in our arms.

Later in that emotional week, on the anniversary of my cardiac arrest, Sue came to meet our little wonder. As she cradled him in her arms, the significance hit her in a way that words couldn't express.

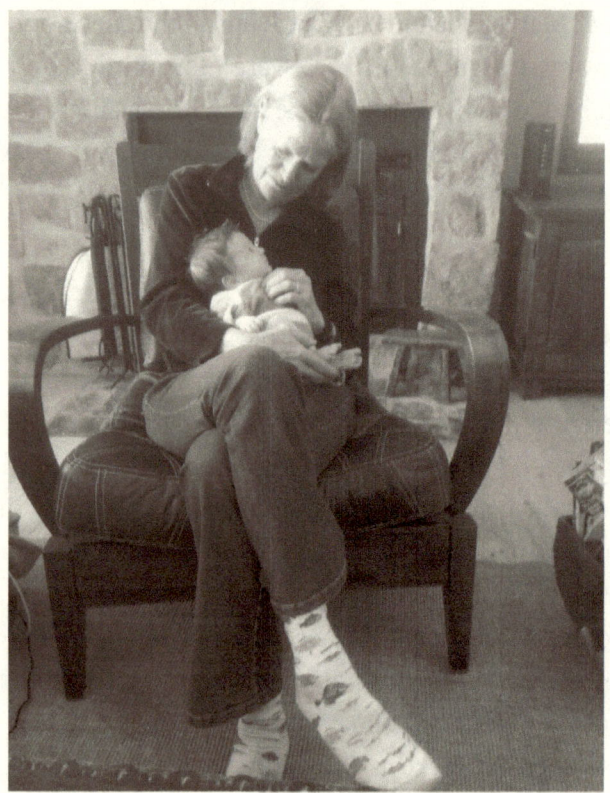

Sue holding Thomas for the first time.

Sue and her sisters never had children. Holding Thomas with his tiny fingers and delicate features was a powerful moment. Tears welled in her eyes, avowing the depth of her emotions.

For Sue, meeting Thomas wasn't just a simple encounter, but an overwhelming connection to a life that wasn't possible without her. It was a reminder that her actions on that fateful day in February 2007 had given rise to something extraordinary. Thomas's existence was proof of the ripple effect of one person's courageous decision.

Sue's role in our lives took on a new meaning at that moment. She didn't need to have her own children to leave a legacy; she had us—her surrogate family. Through her friendship and support with Starting Hearts, she had become a maternal figure to me—a guiding presence in our lives. I lovingly called her my Life Mom, and she embraced her role as Thomas's Life Grandma with open arms.

From that day forward, our bond with Sue deepened, transcending blood to form a connection rooted in gratitude, and a shared incident that began with a single selfless act. In Sue, I found not just a lifesaver, but a lifelong confidante and mentor—someone whose presence would shape our lives in ways we never imagined.

As Grammy and Grandpa bid us farewell and Matt returned to his work routine, I found assurance in the presence of my sister, Margaret. She had always been there when I needed her most; this time was no exception. Her arrival felt like a breath of fresh air, bringing a wealth of experience and wisdom. As a mother of three, Margaret was well-versed in caring for newborns.

During her visit, she shared invaluable maternal knowledge and offered practical advice on everything from mastering the art of swaddling to meticulously cleaning baby bottles. Her calm reassurance instilled confidence in me as I continued to recover and navigate the early days of sleepless nights.

When Margaret's visit ended, so too did the help-filled days I had grown accustomed to. With everyone returning to their responsibilities, I was left to face the world of motherhood on my own. Yet, armed with the lessons Margaret and others had imparted, I approached this new phase with gratitude and a quiet assurance, cherishing their time and wisdom.

Thomas, Charlie, and I sat together in the gentle pendulum of the rocking chair on which my mom once rocked me. A wave of overwhelming emotion washed over me, culminating in tears that flowed freely down my cheeks. In that intense moment, surrounded by the scars of all we had endured, I felt gratitude and contentment settle upon my heart.

With gentle hands, not wanting to disturb either of them, I reached for my phone and captured a snapshot of the scene before me—just me and my boys, bathed in the soft glow of the room. As I gazed at the image, I marveled at the magnitude of blessings in my life. Every trial and tear shed led me to this sacred moment of fulfillment.

In the stillness of that embrace, a quote from Charles Haddon Spurgeon came to mind, resonating with the truth of my journey:

"The longer the blessing comes, the sweeter it will be when it arrives. That which is gained speedily by a single prayer is sometimes only a half-weighted blessing, but that which is gained after a tug and many an awful struggle is a full-weighted and precious blessing. The blessing that costs us the most in prayer will be worth the most."

With those words etched upon my heart, I embraced the preciousness of the present, knowing that every trial had only deepened the richness of the blessings I had received. As we rocked together, I felt an overwhelming sense of peace—a result of enduring faith and undeserved grace.

It was a reminder to acknowledge how far I'd come and to give thanks for all that I had been given.

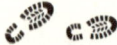

STEP TO REDUCE ANXIETY AND INCREASE HEART HOPE:

Consider the perspective. Focusing on what you do have calms the mind and lifts the heart.

CHAPTER 23
The First Real Baby

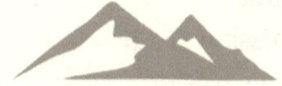

Reflecting on Thomas's existence, I couldn't help but marvel at the extraordinary circumstances that led to his birth. Each event along the way felt like part of a larger design.

Miracles are often met with skepticism, yet when I looked at Thomas, I saw clear evidence of something beyond scientific explanation.

With each passing day, we treasured his presence, recognizing his life as nothing short of a gift. As parents, we were committed to helping Thomas understand the value of life and the incredible path that brought him to us.

People often called Starting Hearts my first baby, and it was. Had I conceived earlier or not experienced that miscarriage five years prior, the organization might never have existed.

By mid-winter, as the Third Annual All You Need is Heart event approached, I felt a surge of energy and enthusiasm. It was a special occasion not only for Starting Hearts but also for Thomas, who was about to make his public debut. With Sue Froeschle in the audience, I stepped on stage and proudly introduced Thomas Froeschle Blake.

It was a moment filled with meaning—a symbol of resilience, hope, and the power of second chances. The event unfolded beautifully, leaving a lasting impression on everyone who attended.

With Alan's leadership and my support, Starting Hearts expanded. We placed more defibrillators, extended our educational programs, diversified funding, and built a strong, committed team.

While preparing for the silent auction, the Tobins met Mare, who was interested in our mission. To bring us all together, the Tobins graciously hosted a dinner at Saddleridge in Beaver Creek.

Mare, a registered nurse, and her husband Bob, a retired general practitioner, radiated warmth and a spirit of service. Bob volunteered with blind skiers, while Mare stayed active working part-time in retail. Their energy was infectious, their interest sincere.

By the end of the evening, they had agreed to help teach classes. The very next day, I ran into them at church—an unexpected affirmation that their involvement was meant to be.

Bob and Mare soon became our lead instructors and fulfilled my vision of training every student in Eagle County—from kindergarten through twelfth grade—reaching over 6,000 children.

We were also fortunate to welcome the experienced Chief McGee, following his retirement from the Vail Fire Department, and Janet, a loving, kind-hearted, seasoned educator and wife of the Jewish Rabbi in Vail. Their experience and standing in the community again elevated the organization and reinforced our reputation as a trusted leader.

With Alan's coordination, our team delivered countless free classes, consistently praised for their professionalism, teamwork, and heart.

Alan continued to exceed expectations, and Starting Hearts thrived.

Thanks to the generosity of the Mowers, Starting Hearts secured its own office—an essential milestone for long-term growth.

Though I stepped back from daily operations, I remained involved at the board level, attending strategic meetings with Thomas in my arms. I was honored with the American Red Cross Humanitarian Hero of the Year award.

Balancing my two roles—mother and mission leader—meant selectively engaging where I was most needed.

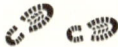

With the organization in excellent hands, I had space to fully embrace caring for Thomas.

For years, I had dreamed of cradling a baby, and the reality exceeded anything I had imagined. The milestones came quickly: soft coos, bright smiles, sitting up, tasting new foods. Though all parents marvel at these moments, Thomas seemed to grow in leaps and bounds.

He slept through the night by eight weeks. By nine months, skipping crawling altogether, he was walking. Friends and strangers alike were astonished to see such a tiny child confidently toddling around.

His first word, "Achie," was his attempt to say Charlie, our dog's name. From ten months old, he pointed to every pup he saw and called them all "Achie," declaring his bond with his furry friend.

The first year with Thomas flew by in an astonishing blur.

As Thomas grew, Matt and I stopped using contraceptives, open to expanding our family. We experienced highs and lows—moments of hope followed by the sorrow of early loss.

After the intense journey that brought us to Thomas, we hesitated to pursue fertility treatments again. We felt profoundly blessed already and weren't eager to invite more complications.

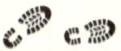

While I relished motherhood, I also missed the independence and purpose that came from contributing professionally. By 2016, the economy was improving, and our family was in a more stable place. I was ready to reengage.

Thomas, full of energy and curiosity, had become a full-fledged toddler. I hired a sitter one day a week so I could return to Starting Hearts with focused energy.

I dedicated eight to twelve hours per week to support our outreach, training, and expansion efforts. Alan welcomed the help as we worked together to educate more citizens and install more defibrillators.

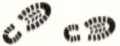

The path that had once been soft with dirt was now covered by leaves. Just as the trail transforms with time, so do our lives, molded by moments that feel larger than ourselves. The seasons remind us that change is inevitable—even when the path is constant. The landscape doesn't ask for permission to evolve, and neither does life. But with each shift comes an opportunity to see the world in a new way. Whether the trail is lined with summer greenery or autumn leaves, it's still the same path, leading us forward.

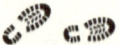

STEP TO REDUCE ANXIETY AND INCREASE HEART HOPE:

Savor the good. Reflect on the blessings in your life and what it took to receive them.

CHAPTER 24
One Fall and Call Away

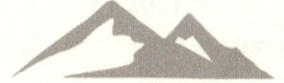

I was in a comfortable groove, the gentle descent prompting me to pick up the pace. The rhythm of my steps felt effortless, almost automatic—until a protruding rock caught my foot, sending me tumbling to the ground. One moment of unsuspecting confidence left me shaken, a jarring reminder of how quickly life can shift without warning.

That same sense of unexpected upheaval defined August 2016. At 6:45 a.m. on Friday the nineteenth, my phone rang. The name "Adrienne" lit up the screen. She would only call this early if something serious had happened. My heart raced. "Hi, Adrienne," I answered cautiously, bracing myself.

Her somber tone confirmed my fears. "I have bad news. . . . "

It was her youngest brother, Drew. He had died in a car accident the night before.

Drew, just eighteen, was her mother's youngest child. He had recently signed to play baseball for Texas Christian University, a Division I college in Fort Worth—a dream he had worked hard to achieve. I remembered him vividly from our family trip to Telluride just months earlier: vibrant, full of life. How could he be gone?

The loss shattered Adrienne's family. The news sent shockwaves through Fort Worth, touching everyone who had cheered him on.

No words could ease their pain, but I offered what I had learned through my suffering—meaning can come from despair. While hope may come in time, nothing could ever replace this loss.

With Thomas still needing constant care, I couldn't travel to attend the funeral. But I needed Adrienne to feel my support. I sent flowers, had food delivered to their home, and tried in every way I could to let her know I was grieving with them.

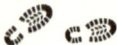

Five days later, on Tuesday, August 23, I was at the Starting Hearts office when my cell phone rang again.

"Lynn? It's Lainie."

Lainie and her husband, Adam, were close friends of Ben and Chelsey. I was surprised to hear from her directly.

"I'm calling to tell you about something that happened during Chelsey's vacation to Lake Powell," she said, her voice trembling.

She went on to recount how Chelsey's two-year-old son had fallen into the water. Without hesitation, she dove in to save him. The physical and emotional toll of the moment overwhelmed her, and she didn't survive.

"Ben's on the way to get the kids," Lainie finished. "I just wanted you to know."

Chelsey couldn't be gone. Just weeks earlier, we had hiked together with our boys. She laughed, talked about faith, and shared her newfound peace. I thanked Lainie through disbelief, unable to say more. The loss struck like lightning—blinding, immediate, and irreversible.

I called Matt to tell him. Then I sat at my desk in silence. The parallels between her death and my brush with mortality were impossible to ignore. My body trembled. I was overcome with grief.

Chelsey had always seemed unbreakable—vibrant, athletic, strong. And now she was gone. I gripped the edge of my desk as tears fell. Her absence was profound. And so was the terrifying realization: no one, no matter how resilient, is immune to death.

News outlets reported her story with the headline: "Mother Drowns in Boating Accident." To me, it was incredibly frustrating. Chelsey didn't drown—she went into cardiac arrest. But the details no longer mattered. Chelsey was gone. It wasn't the time to campaign for cardiac arrest awareness, even though her story highlighted why that awareness was urgently needed.

The grief was overwhelming. I couldn't sleep. I kept thinking about Chelsey—not just as a friend, but as someone who had inspired my work with Starting Hearts. Cardiac arrest had taken her. And I couldn't stop wondering why I survived, and she didn't?

The illusion of control fell apart. I was face-to-face again with the truth I'd encountered in 2007: life is fragile. We are not in control.

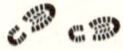

In the weeks after the tragedy, Ben and the children visited. They were in shock, of course, but they were surviving. Despite all they had lost, I was grateful to see some resilience in them.

Adding to the situation's complexity, Ben and Chelsey endured a divorce earlier that year. When Ben returned to Vail two weeks later, he introduced us to Brie—the woman he had been seeing since the separation. From the moment we met, I sensed Brie was someone special.

She exuded warmth and kindness. Her bright blue eyes and gentle smile were instantly disarming. But it was her compassion and openness that made the most significant impression. Watching her with Ben and the children, I couldn't help but feel that this wasn't random. I prayed Brie was part of something planned; that she might bring healing to this grieving family.

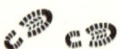

Chelsey's celebration of life took place four weeks later at Mile Hi Church, a large dome-shaped building near her home. It wasn't a traditional church. At the front was a box containing her ashes and her favorite pair of purple running shoes.

A mural representing various world religions—Buddhism, Hinduism, Islam, Judaism, and Christianity—was painted on the walls of the sanctuary. The message was spiritual unity across all beliefs.

But the service left me unsettled. There was no mention of heaven, no affirmations of faith, just vague talk of Chelsey's essence and energy. I believed she was in heaven, and I clung to the memory of our hike and her recent reflections.

Chelsey told me she'd met Brie and blessed her with the job of helping raise her children. More importantly, she said she had been reading the Bible and believed in God. That was enough for me to know that I would see her again.

But it wasn't enough to quiet the unnerving pit in my soul.

I looked into Mile Hi Church's teachings. Their vision of "Oneness revealed" emphasized spiritual empowerment and global enlightenment. It sounded compassionate, but the church's beginnings in a vacuum cleaner store left me questioning its spiritual depth. Still, it spurred me to explore. I wanted to understand what people believed—and why.

After surviving cardiac arrest, faith had become my strength. But I still struggled with questions. Are all religions different trails up the same mountain, leading to the same God?

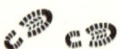

STEP TO REDUCE ANXIETY AND INCREASE HEART HOPE:

Expect pain and heartache. Acceptance is the first step toward healing and future happiness.

CHAPTER 25
Summoning the Courage

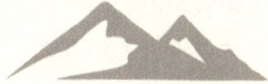

The trail demanded courage I wasn't sure I had, especially after the recent losses. Each step felt heavier, as though the weight of my doubts and grief clung to my feet, threatening to hold me back. Moving forward required more than just physical effort—it demanded the strength to accept the things I could not control and the bravery to keep pressing on.

Infertility remained an uphill climb, but we were grateful for a healthy two-year-old and a new, comfortable home.

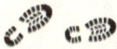

That summer, I made a decision that had weighed on me for years: I stopped taking Adderall. I had long considered the change, but the timing had never felt right. With Adrienne visiting—a friend who accepted me without judgment—I knew the moment had come. I started weaning off, dose by dose, and to my surprise, I no longer felt dependent on it.

But as I released one crutch, I confronted another: my eating disorder. I had hidden this part of me for years, even from Matt. Failing to share my past was imprisonment, keeping me from being myself.

If I wanted true freedom, I had to face it and speak it aloud.

I started by opening up to trusted friends. That vulnerability led to real growth. Sharing my truth wasn't easy, but it brought healing. I was learning to let go of shame and surrender to something greater—to acknowledge my past without letting it define me.

My spirit was urging me to trust that all my circumstances, even the painful ones, had purpose, that my story—full of missteps and unlikely turns—could help someone else. So, I committed to the process.

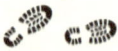

I knew Matt loved me, but telling him filled me with fear. What if he saw me differently? What if this changed us?

One night, while Thomas stayed at my parents' house, Matt and I had a rare date night at Ti Amo—"I love you"—a fitting place for a moment that required so much vulnerability.

Sitting in a quiet corner booth, I gathered my courage and prayed silently. Then I spoke.

"I need to tell you something," I began. "Before we met, I struggled with an eating disorder. I'm okay now, but I feel like I need to tell you."

I didn't go into detail. I didn't need to. Matt reached for my hands.

"How long have you wanted to tell me?" he asked gently. "I wish you had sooner. Lynn, I love you. Nothing will ever change that. I'm just sorry you carried it alone."

His words dissolved my shame. Relief washed over me. Matt's love—committed and strong—wasn't shaken. It wrapped around me, a quiet reassurance that I didn't have to hide anymore.

Through it all, I learned to be thankful—not for freedom from the struggles, but because of them. Every step, every scar, had brought me here.

It was as though a veil had lifted. The girl I once was—before the eating disorder, before Adderall, before the cardiac arrest—had returned. I felt lighter, freer. Restored.

Matt's support and God's grace touched every corner of my life. The weight I'd carried for so long was gone. Finally, trust and surrender were giving me back my joy.

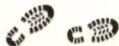

STEP TO REDUCE ANXIETY AND INCREASE HEART HOPE:

Be honest with loved ones. Authenticity deepens connection and builds trust.

CHAPTER 26
There's Always an Obstacle Ahead

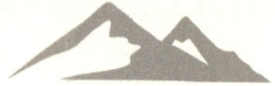

The trail is never smooth or straightforward. After the recent storm, every step presented a new obstacle—a fallen tree to climb over, a jagged rock to avoid, or a slippery root threatening to pull me down. Each challenge mirrored the twists and turns of life, where unexpected setbacks often force us to adjust our course.

On May 31, 2018, life threw me another hurdle. A seemingly innocuous email forwarded by my dad from two national cardiac arrest organizations sent shockwaves through my system. It announced the launch of a Call-Push-Shock campaign—a phrase and program I had painstakingly developed and safeguarded by owning the websites and securing the trademarks. Suddenly, it felt like the storm on the trail had followed me into my mission, presenting yet another challenge to overcome.

As I typed the website, callpushshock.org, my heart sank. To my dismay, I discovered that Starting Hearts no longer owned that domain, or callpushshock.com. Somehow, our ownership had lapsed, leaving our previously protected message vulnerable.

Devastated by the oversight, I reached out to Alan, overwhelmed with disbelief. How could this have happened? After all the effort and purpose poured into this campaign, it felt like a betrayal to see others promoting it as their own.

I had always respected Alan; he handled many responsibilities with competence. But now, our trademarked campaign was in someone else's hands, and I was livid.

Determined to fix it, I urged Alan to contact the organizations responsible. But despite his efforts, they showed little interest in collaborating with Starting Hearts. So, I reached out to the founder myself, a bereaved mother who had lost her son to cardiac arrest.

I shared the history behind Call-Push-Shock and asked that Starting Hearts be recognized as a co-partner. She declined. My devastation confirmed: something I had created and protected had slipped away.

As I fumed at being excluded from something I had worked tirelessly to create, I struggled to reconcile my frustration with the reality unfolding before me. It felt intensely personal, like watching a piece of my heart handed off without acknowledgment. But as the days passed and the initial sting dulled, a quieter truth settled in: the message was reaching more people, saving more lives. That had always been the goal. Even if Starting Hearts wasn't publicly credited, the mission was advancing. And in that truth, I found peace, not because it was easy, but because it was right.

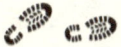

Even with obstacles, Starting Hearts continued to grow. What began as a one-woman mission had become an entire organization, with an executive director, assistant, instructors, and technicians maintaining our network of defibrillators. Our vision expanded into legislative advocacy.

We worked to change Colorado law, which at the time only required schools to accept AEDs if donated. There were no rules for broader public spaces. When we tried placing devices in major stores like Walmart and Home Depot, store managers often declined.

Partnering with local State Representative Dylan Roberts, there was an instant, unspoken connection. Though our experiences were different, our missions were remarkably the same.

Representative Roberts lost his younger brother from complications with diabetes, which became the fire behind his legendary efforts to cap the cost of insulin, a law that expanded nationwide.

I didn't have to explain much to Rep. Roberts; he already understood. When I spoke about cardiac arrest, the lives lost for lack of access, and the urgency that fueled our advocacy, he knew because of his own grief.

For both of us, it was never about politics—it was about mutual convictions to make a meaningful difference in the lives of others.

We championed a bill to expand defibrillator access statewide. Thomas, just four years old, demonstrated how to apply an AED on a manikin and joined me at the Capitol. During our testimony, he impressed lawmakers with his ability at such a young age.

When Governor Polis signed the bill, Thomas and I returned, manikin and defibrillator trainer in hand. We showed him how to use the device—his first time. It may have been a small step, but it was meaningful, and I felt empowered to press on.

The experience led me to consider broader legislation; particularly how cardiac arrest is reported. I envisioned stronger systems to track, understand, and improve survival outcomes across the state.

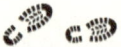

Another opportunity arose when Sue encouraged me to reach out to Susan Ford Bales, daughter of President Gerald and Betty Ford. Vail held deep ties to the Ford family, with landmarks honoring their legacy. Susan had spent time in Vail and was known locally by her Secret Service code name, "Snowflake."

In 2010, at age 52, Susan suffered a cardiac arrest while working out at a gym in Dallas. A nearby doctor saved her life with CPR and a defibrillator. Her story mirrored our mission.

To my surprise and delight, Susan agreed to speak at our February event for free. Like her parents, she felt called to give and use her experiences to help others.

We hosted the event at the Vail Golf Course, a modern venue that honored the Ford family's enduring legacy in our community. As the alpenglow lit the Gore Range in gold, a full moon rose above, welcoming leaders and longtime locals who gathered to support our cause. Susan's speech was heartfelt. She shared her survival from cardiac arrest and honored her mother's heritage with breast cancer advocacy. Her words connected deeply with the audience.

The next morning, as I drove Susan to the airport, I nervously asked if she would continue working with Starting Hearts. She agreed.

Alan and I saw her as the perfect spokesperson for our national campaign, the Save More Lives Challenge. The challenge encouraged people to watch our two-minute training video, practice compressions on a household item, and share it on social media with #SaveMore-Lives. We also launched a petition for legislative support.

Susan agreed to help lead the effort. It felt like righteous alignment.

Meanwhile, Alan pursued a partnership with the national sorority Alpha Phi, beginning with the University of Denver chapter. I was invited to be the keynote speaker at their annual fundraiser.

This time, I approached the speech differently. Using Susan's experienced example, I created a binder to organize my notes, and for the first time, I included details about my eating disorder and Adderall use. I wanted to be honest. To connect. As someone who finds comfort in solitude and quiet reflection, standing on stage was never my natural space. But I knew that vulnerability shared publicly creates deeper connections—making a difference demands visibility, even from those who prefer the background.

Before the event, I noticed girls who reminded me of myself at that age, struggling silently. I hoped my unfiltered story might offer them something.

Afterward, an alum thanked me with tears in her eyes. Weeks later, a six-figure donation and heartfelt note arrived. The funds would support our national campaign.

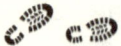

We also began expanding the CARES registry across Colorado. Data from Eagle County showed survival rates 2.5 times higher than the national average, validating our approach. In contrast, Denver ranked among the lowest.

With statewide CARES implementation on the horizon, we helped form a hiring committee to find the right leader. Jillian Moore, with her Colorado Department of Public Health and Environment (CDPHE) background, stood out. She accepted the challenge, and we worked together to assemble a statewide coalition.

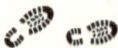

Then Alan brought more news: a respected cardiologist who had supported Starting Hearts agreed to become board chair. I was thrilled—until I learned that his schedule wouldn't allow much involvement. Alan and I would still shoulder most responsibilities.

Despite the disappointment, we moved forward and planned our first board retreat. Rohn, a local attorney and philanthropist, volunteered to moderate.

The retreat was full of reflection, vision casting, and collaboration. And then Rohn said something that stuck with me:

"Every ten years, most nonprofits need a shake-up."

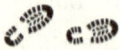

STEP TO REDUCE ANXIETY AND INCREASE HEART HOPE:

Share your story. Your truth may be the encouragement someone else needs.

CHAPTER 27
Leaving My Baby Behind

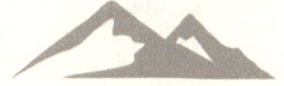

My heart and soul had been poured into the growth and success of Starting Hearts for nearly a decade. Alan and I had made significant strides. As I reflected on our accomplishments, I felt a sense of pride in what we had built together. Alan's leadership had played a critical role in that journey, yet a persistent concern lingered beneath the surface.

Throughout his tenure, I encountered moments of frustration. Each time I raised concerns, Alan would respond with vague reassurances or change the subject. At first, I brushed them off as growing pains, convinced that progress required some compromise. But over time, those moments accumulated.

Everything changed when I learned that an employee had resigned due to internal tensions. I confided in Matt, who looked at me concernedly and said, "You've been dealing with this for too long. It's time to take action."

I reached out to Jim and Sue—my lifesavers and steadfast allies on the board. We knew a tough decision lay ahead. Alan had been vital to Starting Hearts' success, but a change was needed.

Sue, especially, had become more than a board member. She was my rock. Her calm confidence carried a kind of maternal presence—steady, wise, and fiercely loyal. She listened without judgment, reminded me of my strength when I forgot it, and offered both strategic advice and emotional reassurance. Her belief in me never wavered, even when mine did.

Jim and Sue offered to join me for the meeting, but I declined. Over the previous five years, Alan and I had developed an unshakable trust and had navigated every challenge together. I felt that if I was going to deliver this news, it needed to come from me alone.

Still, Sue sensed my unease. Unable to sit on the sidelines, she showed up at my house unannounced. In her hand was a ruby and diamond ring—one she had worn since her mother's passing.

"I want you to have this," she said loyally. "Maybe it'll give you strength in the meeting."

Overcome with emotion, I slipped the ring onto my right hand. Its glimmer reminded me I wasn't alone. It wasn't just a gift—it was a symbol of her commitment to me. I vowed to wear it always.

I summoned my courage and scheduled the meeting with Alan. We sat across from each other in our office, surrounded by the symbols of all we'd built. As gently as possible, I said, "Alan, certain matters have come to light, and we've decided changes are necessary."

At first, he said nothing. His eyes drifted toward the wall where years of milestones were displayed—photos, plaques, a framed mission statement. I recognized the feelings behind his silence. This wasn't just a job to him. Starting Hearts had become his life's work—a legacy.

He made a firm declaration before leaving, and I knew that whatever came next wouldn't be pretty. My heart sank as I realized the magnitude of the situation.

I'd hoped for a quiet, dignified exit. What followed was anything but.

Within days, Alan requested we sign a non-disparagement agreement. I called Jim and Sue immediately. The conversation shifted from mission to mitigation.

The year before, I signed a contract that seemed routine. Within the fine print was tight termination language that effectively locked us into a five-year consulting agreement. He was only one year into the contract and had no intention of stepping down or away. Whether by oversight or optimism, I had committed us to a long-term relationship he wasn't ready to end—and one we weren't fully prepared to continue.

Legal negotiations followed. There were long phone calls and sleepless nights. I never imagined we'd end up here. The very thing I had built to give life was now taking it. Mine. It was a cruel irony I could hardly comprehend.

The deeper we went into the process, the more the emotional cost revealed itself. Jim, once my steadfast ally, grew distant—pulled between loyalty and legality. Alan and I could no longer speak, not even as colleagues. We had built something beautiful together, and now we stood in silence on opposite sides of it.

By early 2020, while the world around me buzzed with energy, I was quietly unraveling. I couldn't sleep. I barely ate. My thoughts spun in circles, caught between grief, resentment, and the fading embers of purpose.

At the same time, hope was rising in our campaign. The Save More Lives Challenge was launching with the support of a national PR firm. There was genuine excitement—TV producers showed interest in our message featuring Susan Ford and reality show stars, Ryan and Trista Sutter. It was the visibility we always dreamed of.

But just as momentum built, the COVID-19 pandemic struck. Headlines changed. Priorities shifted. The spotlight we'd fought so hard for vanished.

And beneath that global chaos, my personal storm continued. Alan wasn't stepping aside. I couldn't ignore the ache of disappointment. Maybe it was easier this way. The rift between us had become irreparable, but I couldn't shake the belief that Alan had been the right person to lead. If he was this determined to stay, then surely, he would carry it forward.

But I also knew something had shifted in me. The fire that had once burned so brightly was now just a flicker. My heart was no longer in the fight.

Starting Hearts had been my first baby—the mission that pulled me from the darkest valley of my life and gave me something to live for. But deep down, I knew the season had shifted. My heart had moved home to Thomas, and personal dreams I had placed on hold.

On March 24, 2020, I sent a farewell email to my contacts. My words were filled with gratitude, but hitting send felt like tearing a piece of my soul away. I was surrendering something I had nurtured for nearly a decade. The grief surprised me. It wasn't just about walking away—it was about letting go of identity, of legacy, of control, of an email I used for a decade.

Then came the silence. Life slowed in lockdown. We were grateful for the nearby trails and the refuge of the mountains, but the stillness made it harder to ignore the desire for focus and control. I tried to stay grounded, but eventually, under the pressures of everything, I returned to Adderall. After nearly two years without it, I consulted my doctor through telehealth and resumed the medication.

That summer, a post appeared in my feed—Starting Hearts was being featured on K-LOVE's *Closer Look*. My heart jumped. I'd listened to K-LOVE for years, even supported with donations. I tuned in with hope.

But as I listened, my chest tightened. Alan and another representative shared the organization's mission, but God was absent from the story. The faith that had shaped it, that had saved me, wasn't mentioned.

I was proud—but I was also heartbroken.

Later, I wrote a gentle note to the producer, thanking them and suggesting a follow-up segment that might share more of the organization's spiritual roots. The response was kind but firm. The story would remain as aired.

And just like that, I exhaled. I had done all I could. My chapter with Starting Hearts had ended.

I released the need to shape its future. No longer guarding the story or controlling its course, I stepped back—trusting the seeds would still bloom, even if I wasn't the one tending the garden anymore.

Whatever came next, I was ready.

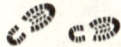

STEP TO REDUCE ANXIETY AND INCREASE HEART HOPE:

Let go. Releasing what you thought was best makes space for what is best.

CHAPTER 28
Long Days, Fast Years

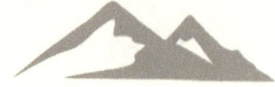

On a seemingly endless day spent at home caring for a young child, my sister-in-law offered a piece of wisdom: "The days are long, but the years fly by." I was too tired to fully grasp its truth in the moment—but she was right. In what felt like a blink, Thomas was heading off to kindergarten in person, his eager face partially hidden behind a mask. It was a small price to pay for a sense of normalcy, especially while much of the world was still confined to remote learning.

Ben and Brie had been through a lot in recent years, and they were finally ready to make their family official. But the pandemic still gripped our lives—restrictions on gatherings, travel limitations, and a cloud of uncertainty over everything. Still, they forged ahead with determination. I admired that about them. Regulations, opinions, and even a global pandemic would not get in their way.

Naturally, I had *Sorry I Party* hats made.

It was the most stunning wedding I'd ever attended—a five-star ranch in Wyoming, surrounded by mountains and sky, with their love shining brightly in the face of lingering grief and the world's chaos. Brie, radiant and poised, addressed the crowd with a perfect blend of humor and wisdom.

"You know what they say," she said with a smile. "If you want to make God laugh, tell Him your plans."

Brie's unexpected thrust into motherhood, stepping into the role for Chelsey's children, was the last thing she had planned. Her heartfelt vows, filled with love and promise, left no eye dry. In that moment, she became their mom in every way that mattered. And yet, somehow, despite it all, she made it look effortless.

Their union was more than a celebration of love; it was a powerful reminder that something beautiful can be born even from tragedy.

With Thomas settled in school, I embraced a sliver of freedom. I deepened friendships, spent time in nature, hiked, and skied, returning to the mountains that had long been my sanctuary. Though I remained involved in advocacy, I had scaled back. Jillian had taken the lead as Colorado's CARES coordinator, and I continued to support her from a seat on the state's data committee. My mission lived on, even as I approached it at a more measured pace.

Just as quickly as it began, the kindergarten year ended, ushering in summer once again. Life's seasons were flying by.

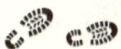

Living in a ski town creates a transient, tightly knit community. Friends come and go, leaving lasting marks. Close friends from Matt's college years were moving away after two years in Vail. To say goodbye, we planned to host a farewell party for about seventy guests.

To help manage the logistics, I hired Loida, a talented caterer and a connection from church. After weeks of dry summer weather, rain poured on the event day, and we scrambled to move everything under a tent. Loida adapted gracefully, helping the party run smoothly despite the last-minute interruptions.

After the event, Loida remarked at the comfort she felt in our home and asked if she could stay with us for two weeks in July between catering jobs. I was grateful for her help and agreed.

Several weeks later, tragedy struck again. On June 30, 2021, my mom called with a trembling voice: Addison, Pastor Craig's eldest daughter, had died in a car accident involving seven girls. She was the only one who didn't survive.

Our church community was devastated. How could this happen to such a faithful family?

I called Adrienne immediately. She, too, knew the pain of losing a sibling. Adrienne had visited The Vail Church many times, often drawing strength and inspiration from Pastor Craig's heartfelt messages. If anyone would understand the significance of this moment and want to know, it was Adrienne. She had come a long way since Drew's passing—even founding a baseball tournament that helps fund college tuition for young athletes.

As plans for Addison's memorial took shape, Loida reached out from Florida, offering to help coordinate meals once she returned. The church asked if we could host family members attending the service in our apartment, but I had to decline—Loida was staying with us.

Loida arrived late one night and settled in easily. We exchanged brief greetings at church that Sunday. A few days later, on July 21, she messaged to say she had tested positive for COVID. She would quarantine in the apartment.

Days passed with no contact. I gave her space, but by July 29, I became worried. A spoiled cooler at the top of the stairs and her lack of response alarmed me. I texted: "If I don't hear from you in one hour, I'll call 911."

No reply.

With my parents caring for Thomas, I called emergency services. A police officer arrived and entered the apartment. Minutes later, he returned with the words I feared: "Your concerns are confirmed."

Loida had passed away, likely three days prior. The shock was immense. Had Thomas wandered downstairs earlier, it would have been traumatic. Now we had to face the unimaginable reality of death in our home.

The coroner, clad in black rubber overalls, carefully removed the body. Because of the COVID risk, no autopsy would be performed.

We were instructed to remove furniture and sanitize the space. That evening, stunned and grieving, Matt and I tried to decompress over dinner. I informed my parents, who shared the news with the leaders filling in for Pastor Craig.

The next morning at church, the outpouring of support was overwhelming. Women from the Cracked Pots group offered to pack Loida's belongings. Others removed her car and disposed of contaminated items. Our new housekeeper stepped in with discretion and professionalism.

And yet, a haunting lingered.

At night, I lay awake, staring at the ceiling. I kept replaying the scene—the quiet apartment, the spoiled cooler, and the police officer's face when he returned from downstairs. Something inside me felt changed. I couldn't stop wondering: Did something spiritual happen here? Was Loida still lingering in some way? Her friend had said she was grateful Loida passed in a peaceful place, but peace was not what I felt.

Later that evening, I curled up next to Matt on the couch. The TV flickered silently in front of us, but we weren't watching.

"I keep thinking about her," I whispered. "She died just below us. Alone. I can't stop imagining what she must've felt in those last moments."

Matt didn't speak right away. He reached for my hand. "I've been thinking about it too," he said. "It's heavy. I just . . . I don't know what to say to make it feel better."

I sighed. "It's not just her death. It's everything it brought up. I thought I'd processed my own mortality, but this dredges it up again."

He looked over, his eyes reflecting concern. "What questions?"

"Like, what happens after we die? Did she know? Was she afraid? Could we have prevented it?"

Matt gently scratched my back to provide comfort. "I don't have all the answers. As we know, death is a part of life—and somehow, we need to move on."

His words landed gently, but the disturbance remained.

The days that followed were heavy with mental and literal fog. I couldn't bring myself to go downstairs. I wondered if our home was still ours—or if her passing had somehow transformed it into something spooky. The air felt thick, and I longed for sunlight, clarity, and a sign that all was well. As the rain poured for days, my anxiety increased, and I was convinced it was time for us to move. I longed for the clouds to part and prayed for sunshine and a sign of hope.

Three days later, Matt called me outside just before sunset. The rain had stopped, and across the valley stretched two vibrant rainbows. It was a sign. My heart lifted.

That evening, I told Matt I needed to bring life to the space if we were to stay. By chance, a neighbor mentioned a client, Monica, a heart surgeon whose home had burned down, who needed a temporary place to live. Monica was undeterred by the apartment's history and would move in with her daughter in September.

Soon after, Matt's parents visited to keep Thomas while Matt and I took a quick trip to Mexico. It was exactly what we needed, something about water meeting land has a way of resetting perspectives. In the Riviera Maya, we found relief from one of the strangest and most disturbing moments we'd ever endured.

Reflecting on the sequence—Loida's help, her stay, her passing, her memorial—I asked myself if we were placed in her life for a reason. Perhaps God had orchestrated it all.

Her death, along with Addison's, brought mortality back into sharp focus. I couldn't stop thinking about how fleeting life truly was.

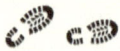

The Book of Psalms often speaks of life's brevity, calling it a vapor, a breath, a shadow. I once heard an analogy—its source now lost to me—about being handed stacks of blank sheets of paper at birth, one for each day of life. Each page represents a new chance to live purposefully. By night, the page is gone, never to return.

Carrying that concept forward, I created a "Days of Your Life" jar—30,000 slips of biodegradable paper, each one symbolizing a single day in an average lifespan. I keep the jar next to the kitchen sink, near the window where the morning light first breaks through.

Each morning, or whenever I remember, I remove paper—sometimes letting it drift away in the breeze, and other days clasping it as if it were a small sacred token. This simple act has become a ritual, a mindful pause to acknowledge another day granted to me.

Our time on this earth is counted and ticking by. But in these small slips of paper, I find meaning in each day—a reason to reflect, and to appreciate.

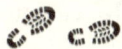

STEP TO REDUCE ANXIETY AND INCREASE HEART HOPE:

Honor each day. Appreciate its purpose and time in the scheme of life.

INSTRUCTIONS FOR CREATING
A "DAYS OF YOUR LIFE" JAR

Find a Jar
Reuse a clean glass or plastic jar with a lid.

Prepare Your "Days"
Use dissolving confetti or cut biodegradable paper into tiny pieces, approximately 25,000-30,000 pieces for an entire lifespan.

Mark One Year
Count out 365 pieces, one to represent each day of a year.

Measure a Scoop
Use a tablespoon to measure how many pieces fill one scoop.

Build Your Lifespan
Multiply that scoop by the number of years you expect to live beyond today (for example, 32 scoops if you're 50 and estimate living to 82).

Fill Your Jar
Drop each measured scoop into the jar until it's complete.

Display Your Reminder
Place the jar somewhere you'll regularly see it.

Honor Each Day
Daily (or whenever you think of it), remove and discard the paper—blow it to the wind, burn it safely, recycle it—then take a moment to reflect on the gift and purpose of the day.

CHAPTER 29
The One I Waited For

During my time at Starting Hearts, I struggled with not having a personal connection to someone whose life I had directly saved. Though our programs had improved survival rates, I longed for a face—a story—that would validate the mission.

That changed one afternoon at the baseball fields during Thomas's last game of the season. I ran into a mom friend who I hadn't seen since Addison's memorial. As I thanked her for bringing popsicles to celebrate the team, she shared something that stopped me cold.

She told me a man had survived cardiac arrest at E-Town, a local restaurant. His girlfriend performed CPR while a patron used the PulsePoint app to locate a defibrillator—one I had helped install. The man saved was Doug Schwartz, the restaurant's owner. It was the moment I had been waiting for.

That night, I was overwhelmed with a rush of emotion unlike any other: relief, joy, and a profound sense of fulfillment. The work I'd done—every meeting, every training, every challenge—had saved a life.

The next morning, I hiked to process the news. That day's reading, 1 Corinthians 9, spoke of giving oneself to save others. It confirmed what I already knew: the years of commitment had not been in vain.

Soon after, I learned Doug had two sons at Thomas's school. I pulled up the student directory, and sure enough, his number was right there. Part of me wanted to call immediately, to hear his voice, to confirm. But I also understood what he'd been through. Recovery, both physical and emotional, takes time. So I waited a few months before contacting him.

I felt grateful—this wasn't just an answered prayer; it was an intricate connection of purpose, patience, and promise.

Reaching that emotional peak was the top of a mountain I had been climbing for years. Every rejection, every doubt—all of it was worth it, each one leading to my fulfilled mission.

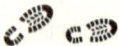

That fall, I stepped into the role of classroom mom and began planning an event for Thomas's school. But my attention quickly turned to an urgent challenge: Colorado's CARES Registry.

The two-year funding from CARES National had ended. Participating agencies couldn't sustain it, and Jillian's role as registry coordinator was eliminated. Still, Jillian volunteered to keep it running.

Though no longer involved with Starting Hearts, I was still involved with the CARES committee and worked closely with Jillian. Together, we approached now Senator Roberts and advocated for the registry's survival.

Eagle County Paramedic Services—the same agency that had once saved me—stepped in to serve as a fiscal sponsor. Encouraged by their support, I began drafting legislation to create a cardiac arrest office within CDPHE. The office would oversee staff, fund the registry, and mandate reporting of out-of-hospital cardiac arrests.

Jillian and I worked relentlessly to keep the bill alive, but we needed someone with real influence—someone who could help us secure the endorsements necessary for it to pass.

Then, as fate would have it, an email arrived from John Seward, a lobbyist interested in helping support our bill. John's family name was forever tied to bold, visionary leaps. His ancestor, William H. Seward, had orchestrated the 1867 purchase of Alaska—a move widely ridiculed at the time as "Seward's Folly," but one history would prove to be a stroke of genius.

In our own way, we were carrying forward that same legacy: believing in possibilities others couldn't yet see—and doing whatever it took to bring them to life.

John became an active champion and a crucial ally with expertise navigating the Capitol.

Our first draft of the bill faced immediate resistance, especially from hospitals and coroners opposed to mandatory reporting. With John's help, we revised it to focus on achievable goals. After gaining the support of agencies and lobbyists, our proposal was ready.

It was an exhausting but empowering process that taught me that change doesn't happen without a little give. It takes persistence, strategy, and the right people in your corner.

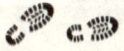

In December, after giving Doug several months to recover from his cardiac arrest, I finally dialed his number. My heart pounded as I waited for him to pick up. When he answered, his voice was steady and kind.

"Hi Doug," I said, "You don't know me, but I just had to call. My name is Lynn. I'm a fellow cardiac arrest survivor and the founder of Starting Hearts."

There was a brief pause, and then his voice lit up with emotion.

"You're the one who helped put the defibrillator outside of E-Town, right? I've been wanting to thank you. That device saved my life."

He was gracious and eager to connect. We spoke like old friends and made plans to meet in person the following week.

When we met at a coffee shop, the recognition and connection were instant. We found a quiet table among the morning crowd and exchanged survival stories. I shared how faith and belief in something greater had helped me find peace after my cardiac arrest. Doug listened kindly, then nodded and clarified, "I'm not really spiritual." He wasn't dismissive—just honest. I left it at that, respecting his stance while still feeling the significance of our convergence. I emphasized how powerful his testimony could be. Doug agreed to speak in support of our bill. We snapped a photo to mark the moment.

That meeting was just the beginning—the first of many

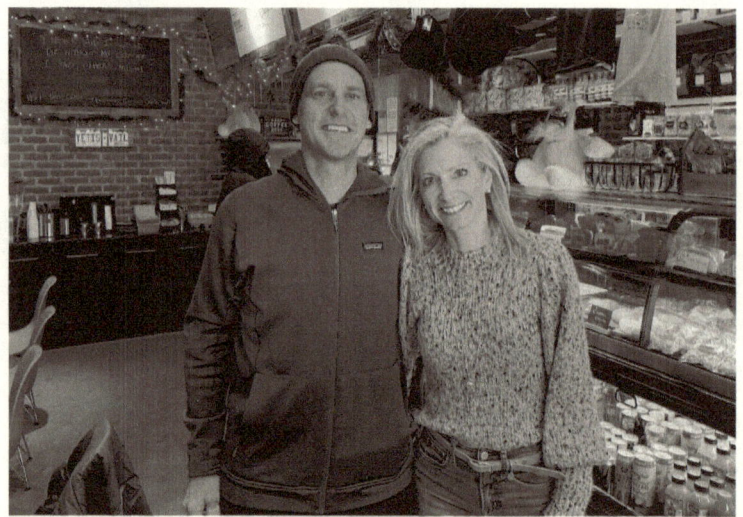

Meeting Doug for the first time.

conversations that would blossom into a sincere friendship. Doug and I spoke periodically, checking in on each other as survivors.

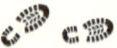

The legislative road was tough. Establishing laws—even when it's logical—invites opposition. Some criticisms felt personal, bringing me to tears.

One evening, a supporter called with encouragement: "This is just like a Hallmark movie." I smiled, remembering all the heart-warming tales Gammy and I had watched together. That comparison lifted me.

Thomas got involved this time, too. He demonstrated CPR and even testified with a heartfelt speech. With John's guidance and liberal support, the bill passed. Coverage was minimal—only CBS 4 aired the story—but seeing Thomas perform CPR on television was enough.

Our work did catch the attention of the AHA, which invited Doug and me to be featured in their scientific statement released alongside the International Liaison Committee on Resuscitation. The chance to help raise global awareness was exhilarating. We were also honored to be included in CARES' national report.

Despite the recognition, public attention was muted. Still, the impact was real. Thirteen years of effort had led to a moment of measurable change.

On June 1, 2022, Governor Jared Polis signed the bill into law. I felt an overwhelming sense of closure.

With advocacy behind me, I finally had room to breathe. What was next? I wasn't sure. So, I returned to the trail.

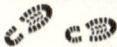

Then, a paramedic friend pushed me to run for the Eagle County Paramedic Services board—the agency that saved my life.

The idea felt daunting. But it was also a perfect full-circle moment. It wasn't just a role, but a chance to serve those who had served me.

I ran, prepared, and waited. Out of nine candidates, I was one of three elected. It was more than validation—it was affirmation that my journey, with all its twists and turns, had meaning.

Board service brought new challenges and growth. It reminded me that even after reaching one peak, there's always another ahead.

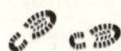

STEP TO REDUCE ANXIETY AND INCREASE HEART HOPE:

Don't stop believing. Hope gets you through, even in the lowest moments.

CHAPTER 30
Life Is Never Boring

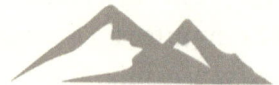

By now, I'd spent a little time on the mountain. And even though I hiked the same trail day after day, each ascent felt different, like the surrounding atmosphere had subtly shifted, revealing something new. It's the same trees, the same incline, the same dirt path, yet somehow, it never feels the same. Each step brings a fresh view, even though it is the same place.

The trail moves with the rhythm of my heart. Whether I'm wrestling with a problem, lost in question, full of gratitude, or simply caught in a song, nature seems to respond—offering clarity, perspective, or some small reminder of how far I've come. It's not just a path; it's part of me.

That's the beauty of it—the expectation stays the same, but the experience is always new. Belief in God is like that. Some say faith requires dull repetition: reading the same literature, praying the same prayers, walking the same spiritual path. But routine doesn't mean lifelessness.

Quite the opposite. Most recently, life has been full of twists—fulfilled predictions, strange encounters, full-circle moments, shifting standards, and unexplainable fulfillment. Belief in something bigger hasn't dulled my life—it's made it a wild, meaningful ride, offering more than I ever expected.

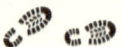

With the new school year and ski season approaching, Thomas's skills on the slopes were advancing quickly, leaving me behind. It was a bittersweet realization—pride in his growth mixed with nostalgia for the days when I could keep up—a reminder of how fast time passes and how quickly everything evolves.

Matt and Thomas are avid football fans and rarely miss a televised game, so it was surprising that we weren't watching on January 2, 2023. But my phone lit up with messages from people I knew, all asking the same thing: Had I seen what happened?

That night during Monday Night Football, the world watched Buffalo Bills safety #3, Damar Hamlin, collapse after a routine play. He stood up, adjusted his helmet, and suddenly dropped, motionless. Medical teams rushed to him, performing CPR and using a defibrillator for nearly twenty minutes before he was transported by ambulance.

As I watched the replays and listened to the commentators' growing concern, a strange calm washed over me: certainty. I knew he would survive. The swift response—immediate CPR and defibrillation—gave him a fighting chance.

It was later confirmed he had suffered cardiac arrest because of a rare event known as commotio cordis—when a sudden, blunt impact to the chest disrupts the heart's rhythm. As the world held its breath waiting for updates, media outlets and friends reached out to ask for my thoughts.

One of them was our dear old friend, Devon. I told him, candidly, "I've been waiting for this moment for fifteen years." I had always known it would take a high-profile event to bring cardiac arrest into the spotlight. And yet, I couldn't help feeling frustrated. After all the work we had done in Colorado—new legislation, defibrillator access, public education—it hadn't received the recognition it deserved.

Devon, now a freelance journalist for major publications, saw the potential. He offered to pitch the story. With his support, I felt hopeful that the awareness we'd been working toward for so long might finally reach a broader audience.

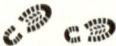

A month later, Matt's parents came to visit. His dad, David, was eager to get on the mountain. After taking a few runs, he, Thomas, and I planned to break for lunch at Two Elk restaurant.

Getting there required a long uphill skate. As we caught our breath, I joked, "That'll get your heart going!"

Moments later, as we reached the lodge, I saw a man collapse in the snow.

I stopped to see if he arose. The scene was all too familiar. His companions stood frozen.

"Call ski patrol! Start CPR! Get a defibrillator!" I shouted, rushing to take off my skis.

No one was acting. Again, I shouted, "call ski patrol and get the defibrillator!"

Leaving my skis and poles behind, I ran toward him, heart pounding, preparing to start compressions—my adrenaline was so high, I feared I might be the one who needed help.

As I approached, there were obvious signs of distress. His goggles were crooked, pressing his nose to his face, preventing breathing. His arms flailed to the side. No movement. No response.

I hesitated, deciding whether to move his goggles to clear the airway, or unzip his jacket for more precise compressions. His body jerked. I questioned if it was an agonal breath, a common reflex during cardiac arrest.

Seconds later, he sat up. Adjusted his goggles. Acting as if nothing happened.

In disbelief, I asked and explained, "Are you okay?" He replied with a puzzled look. "You collapsed. I was about to perform CPR and ski patrol has been called to help."

To make sense of the situation, he said, "I had an implanted defibrillator placed several months ago."

That explained the jump in his body. His ICD delivered a shock to restart his heart. "Wow, you sure are lucky—that device just saved your life!"

Thankfully, I didn't have to administer care—to put into practice everything I'd spent years teaching. Yet, even with all my confidence and knowledge, I still questioned the response in the moment of surprise.

For the first time, I witnessed an ICD working in real life—and for once, it wasn't mine. Relief and adrenaline left me shaking.

Later that spring, during my weekly volunteer shift at Vail Health, I entered a room with a familiar presence. I squinted in the dim light, unsure.

It was Jim Spell, the firefighter, who had helped save my life and served as a mentor for so many years.

I approached with a smile. "Hi, my name is Lynn. I'm a volunteer with the hospital—and I have chocolate chip cookies and lemonade. Would you like some?"

He didn't seem to recognize me but responded quietly, "I'm not hungry, but I'd love to see what you brought."

I wheeled the cart into his room and couldn't hold back: "Jim, it's Lynn Blake."

His face lit up.

He stood to hug me, and we talked for thirty minutes. He shared about a book he was working on, *Star Valley*, and his time in seminary—how he'd studied theology to avoid the draft and later worked in religious broadcasting that he hadn't believed in.

He called himself a spiritual agnostic.

As we spoke, I felt it wasn't a coincidence. "Jim," I said, "this encounter is intentional."

When the nurse came in, I held back tears. I explained how much he meant to me—how he not only saved but also changed my life. She handed me a tissue.

Before I left, Jim revealed he was battling stage 4 inoperable cancer. It might be the last time I saw him. But if it was, I was thankful for our last farewell.

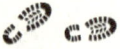

A few weeks later, I was invited to attend an AHA symposium—the first of its kind in over two decades—revived after Damar Hamlin's collapse.

I always believed it would take a highly visible event to ignite critical awareness for cardiac arrest—and I was right. When his incident was broadcast live to millions, everything changed. Remarkably, Damar not only survived but made a full recovery and was now using his voice to champion the cause that had so desperately needed him all along.

The resulting surge in CPR training, defibrillator access, and public conversation was unlike anything the industry had ever seen.

Finally, the cause had a face.

The symposium brought together one hundred global leaders in cardiac arrest advocacy. Sitting among them, I felt honored—and overwhelmed.

The conversations were technical, and I hesitated to speak up. I followed up in writing, sharing three core ideas: definition, data, and dollars.

Cardiac arrest should have an official definition. Without clear causes and consistent classifications, it will continue to be misreported as a heart attack or simply an "unknown cause of death." Until we collect comprehensive data, we cannot fully understand the scope of the problem or identify real solutions.

The cause also needs resources. Despite its devastating impact, cardiovascular disease—and cardiac arrest in particular—receives only a fraction of the funding allocated to other leading causes of death.

Language matters too. "AED" should be replaced with clearer terms, like "defibrillator" or even "Heart Starter."

Most of all, we need to make CPR less intimidating. I proposed a campaign using the C-P-R acronym: "C-Call" to engage help.

"P-Pump" keeps the heart beating. And, "R-Restart" replaces the word "shock," to offer hope instead of fear.

I came back to the most significant opportunity to improve survival rates lies in the residential setting.

Defibrillators should be over-the-counter, without prescription, under $300, covered by insurance, and in every home. Once that happens, all the mapping and costly innovative solutions like drone delivery become irrelevant. Until then, neighborhoods, small businesses, and even individual families need to pool resources to purchase defibrillators for public access.

The response was positive. And I left the symposium inspired and ready to keep pushing.

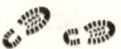

Some of life's most defining changes are subtle: a stranger's offhand comment, a passing headline, a friend's new obsession. Each encounter leaves an imprint. Over time, I noticed a shift—not in myself, but everywhere around me. The pace was quickening. People on TV, and that I knew, were shrinking sizes. And the promotional messages were becoming even more relentless.

The standards for health, beauty, and worth were growing increasingly extreme. After years of working to maintain a balanced and sustainable lifestyle, I had finally made peace with the natural changes of aging—an extra few pounds, softening skin, deeper laugh lines. These were signs of a life well lived, not problems to fix.

But just as I reached acceptance, the goalposts moved.

Today, the line between wellness and vanity is nearly invisible. The rise of injectables, weight-loss drugs, and constant media exposure has reshaped not only how we view others, but also how we see ourselves. It's no longer just celebrities—it's men and women, friends, associates, even the 20- to 30-year-olds who are far from needing intervention. The directive is clear: don't just be healthy, be perfect.

There's no denying that medications assist countless, myself included. In fact, they will spare many from the self-inflicted pain I endured for years, reshaping how we classify and treat eating disorders altogether.

But there's a difference between treatment and altering ourselves in the name of health. What concerns me is the underlying message that it's never enough to be ourselves.

Anyone who has watched TV with me has heard my diatribe about the machine behind it all: the pharmaceutical industry and its relentless advertisements. The U.S. is one of only two countries that allow direct-to-consumer drug advertising. Billions are spent convincing us we're not enough—so we'll spend more trying to improve. Medications meant for serious treatment are marketed like lifestyle upgrades, sandwiched between sitcoms, news, and sports. What's the point of having doctors if we're expected to self-diagnose from a thirty-second commercial?

Consider the dollars wasted, money that could lower the actual cost of medical care, instead of making us feel sick.

This isn't just about medicine—it's about messaging.

So here we are—chasing the latest trends, tweaking, trimming, tightening. One day it's this, tomorrow it's that. The only constant is change.

And with every shift, it remains the same old trail of life—but with more impossible standards. Even grounded in gratitude and wellness, I still feel the tug of unrelenting pressure. Because in today's culture, peace with yourself is no longer possible.

Decades ago, Bob Marley captured the problem: *people are rejected for being real, while those who are fake are being celebrated.* That contradiction feels more relevant than ever today.

The pace of change in our world is beyond comprehension. From unrealistic beauty standards to scientific breakthroughs, the rate of evolution is disorienting. I can't help but wonder what life will look like in 200 years. As we decode the genome and borrow traits from other species—like the insect's ability to freeze and return to life—it's not far-fetched to imagine a future of cryopreservation and bioengineering so advanced we can't fathom.

By then, race and ethnicity may merge into a singular, global identity. Technology and synthetic enhancements will probably touch every corner of human existence. Artificiality may become the norm. We may forget what it means to simply *be*—to live in a body, in a place, in a moment untouched by code or chemicals.

And honestly? I don't want to see that world.

Because I wouldn't belong in it.

What I believe will endure is nature.

The earth, in all its magnificence, holds connections that transcend time and human advancements. The trail doesn't care how flawless your skin is or how optimized your DNA might be. It only asks that you come as you are. With every step, it grounds us—reminding us we are part of something older, wilder, and far more enduring than anything we could ever design.

Years pass. Seasons change. And still, the mountains remain.

Under a canopy of pine or along a wind-worn ridge, I return to what is real. With every hike, I remember: *This is what lasts. This is what matters.*

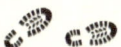

Life is not about walking a rigid, unchanging path—it's about embracing our evolution, finding purpose in the unexpected, in new and dynamic ways.

I've learned to embrace life's pleasures—whether sharing a cocktail, seeking support through prescribed stimulants, or experiencing moments of transcendence. These choices don't conflict with my spirituality; they deepen my understanding of life and perception.

This connection comes alive most vividly on familiar trails. The physical and spiritual intertwine as the sweat on my brow meets a sweeping view, or the stillness of the woods quiets my soul. Each hike reminds me that divinity is woven into every moment—both the ordinary and the extraordinary.

Life is rarely boring. It's a sacred adventure of discovery, where each step calls me to trust the path and One guiding it. No matter how familiar the journey, there's always something new inviting us to grow, explore, and find wonder.

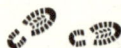

STEP TO REDUCE ANXIETY AND INCREASE HEART HOPE:

Build your identity on timeless principles. It is impossible to maintain the standards of an everchanging world.

CHAPTER 31
It All Ends the Same Way

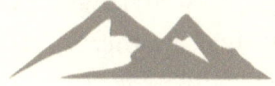

The end of the trail eventually arrives for all of us. It marks the conclusion of this story—my story, your story, every story. It's a truth as inevitable as the rising sun and the changing seasons.

As I set out on this brisk morning hike, the scenery seemed tranquil at first glance. The sky was a brilliant shade of blue, and the sun peeked over the mountain, casting its rays across the snow. But beneath this serene façade, a biting chill lingered in the air, and the wind whipped around me with relentless force.

I resisted the urge to drown out my thoughts with music, choosing instead to embrace the silence.

The year began with a string of interruptions. Starting with a routine visit to Dr. Prager when the ICD interrogation revealed another fractured lead. Since it was the atrial wire again, I postponed the repair until the end of ski season. From there, I went from celebrating Valentine's Day with Sue to a February break trip with Thomas to Jackson, Mississippi, where we visited my ninety-eight-year-old grandmother, Gammy. Though confined to her chair, she remained sharp.

Birthdays are usually low key for me, but this year felt significant. Some of our closest friends had invited us to join their table at the Carpenters Ball, a Habitat for Humanity fundraiser. Dressed in

Western attire, we looked forward to an evening of philanthropy and fun to support local housing initiatives.

Excitement filled the room as the auctioneer presented a bottle of champagne. On a whim, I started the bidding—and won.

Seated beside me, my dear friend Erin handed me a birthday card. The heartfelt words and drawings from her and her daughters touched me deeply. The champagne flowed, laughter filled the room, and the night felt light and joyful. Then, another friend approached with warm wishes—but her expression shifted as she delivered unexpected news.

"Happy birthday," she said kindly, her voice laced with sympathy. "I'm sorry; I know it's been a tough day."

Confused, I replied, "Yeah, Matt's been swamped, but that's nothing new. I enjoyed a hike this morning and was looking forward to celebrating tonight."

Her face softened. "Oh no, Lynn, I thought you knew. Doug Schwartz passed away today."

My heart sank. "What?!" I gasped. Shocked by the bomb that was dropped. "But I thought he was recovering well, being monitored . . . everything was looking up."

Sadness overtook me. Doug had survived cardiac arrest because of the defibrillator I had placed. We had grown close. I attended his "re-birthday" parties—annual celebrations to acknowledge the day he was saved. Each time, I felt honored to be there, to witness the life he was living so fully.

His death felt like a gut punch—a direct blow to the heart of my life's mission.

Just two weeks earlier, Doug had texted me shortly after my re-birthday.

"Hi Lynn, I hope you're well. I was thinking about you and Matt on Valentine's Day, wishing you love and happiness! I'm in Denver now on the heart transplant list. Things have progressed quickly."

"I'm in good spirits and excited for the chance at good long-term health! I'll send a CaringBridge link for updates."

I followed his updates, full of optimism, as he waited for a donor. He and his girlfriend, Shelly, who had performed CPR during his cardiac arrest, married in the hospital, exchanging rings made of foil. Then, there was an update about his successful transplant. Subsequent posts about his positive recovery followed. Four days passed without a new post, but I assumed things remained steady. I had intended to send flowers and a note—meant to—but life got in the way.

And now he was gone.

Beneath the noise and clinking glasses, grief swelled silently within me. Erin and Matt, seated on either side, knew the depth of my connection to Doug. They didn't need to say anything. Their understanding presence offered the space I needed to grieve in the middle of a public moment.

The ride home with Matt was mostly quiet, the air thick with unspoken sorrow. Though Doug was no longer here, the bond we shared—and the work I carried out in his honor—would never fade. His light will remain, illuminating my path forward.

What made it harder to accept was Doug's uncertain spiritual stance. I searched the night sky for a sign that his soul had found peace.

The next day, I called my mom to share the news. I told her how deeply it troubled me. She reminded me I had done my part—I had shared my beliefs with him. The rest, she said, was between him and the Almighty.

Still, another loss weighed on my heart—the memorial service for Steve Zuckerman, a paramedic, ski patroller, and Mountain Rescue volunteer who had supported Starting Hearts from the beginning. Steve and his family helped with the HeartRod project, conducted trainings, and even hung our homemade Starting Hearts banner at the Beaver Creek World Cup ski races.

Two weeks prior, I received the notice from Eagle County Paramedics that Steve suffered a cardiac arrest while rescuing a skier trapped in an avalanche. Despite efforts to revive him, he was pronounced dead at the scene.

My mom had known Steve, too. She cited his Jewish faith and suggested something that unsettled me: because he didn't believe in Jesus as the promised Messiah, he might not be in heaven.

I challenged her. "You told me Jewish people are God's chosen ones. Are you saying Steve isn't in heaven?"

Her response was unwavering: she believed that faith in Jesus was required.

That belief has never sat right with me.

Where my mom finds comfort in strict interpretation of the Bible, I find room for mystery. I believe God leaves space for the questions we can't answer—*How does one God connect with every person? How does one get to heaven? Who created God?*

To me, faith isn't having all the answers. It's holding the ambiguity with trust, not fear. I urged my mom to stay open-minded to the unknowns, reminding her that no one truly knows what happens after death. I suggested to my mom that maybe, in that ultimate moment, everyone sees and accepts God. Maybe death is not the end but a door; on the other side, there's understanding and acceptance.

She paused, then admitted, "Anything is possible."

We don't know what lies beyond, but I can't help but imagine that death holds something greater than what we experience here. We enter this world without choice, and many of us find it a remarkable existence. Just as surely as we enjoyed this life, shouldn't we expect the same of the next?

Our fear and unease with death stem from our lack of control over it. It often arrives with pain, and its aftermath leaves a lasting ache in the hearts of those left behind.

That night, at Steve's memorial service, his daughter shared touching memories, including teaching CPR together with Starting Hearts. Her words stirred something deep in me.

Afterward, the crowd honored him with a snowcat procession and fireworks over Beaver Creek Mountain, where he had served on the ski patrol. It was a fitting tribute to a man whose life was rooted in rescue, service, and family.

Reflecting on both Steve and Doug, I felt a quiet peace. Our paths had crossed for a reason. They had marked my life, and in turn, I had marked theirs.

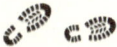

In the weeks that followed, anxiety crept in. Life and death were pressing in on me again. The time had come to address the fractured wire. I was terrified. Another lead extraction meant another high-risk surgery—another chance my heart would be stopped.

I didn't want this to be the end.

Thomas was still young. Matt needed me. But if I didn't make it, someone else would take care of them. That thought—letting go of my family—nearly crushed me.

I stepped onto the trail and prayed—not for rescue, but for reassurance, for some sign that life still lay ahead.

At the familiar turnaround point—a small bridge over the creek—Rosie Sue, my latest ruby-red Cavalier King Charles, sniffed at her pee-mails as I looked up and saw it: a freshly cut tree stump. Something about the trunk held my gaze. Maybe it was the morning light casting a glow around it or the freshness of the cut.

My eyes evaluated its rings. To the left of the center, a deep scar ran through—a jagged interruption in its otherwise smooth cut.

I saw my own life represented; a clear dividing line etched into its rings. That deep wound marked my cardiac arrest, the moment my world split in two: the life I had before, and the one I had been given after.

In some mystical way, that stump was me.

Assessing the rings, I estimated about twenty-seven before the mark—my cardiac arrest—and fifty after. The tree had lived long after its wound.

So would I.

Whether or not it was divine, that stump was my sign. I felt it in my soul. God's messages don't always come in thunder. Sometimes, they come in silence, in subtle things. You just have to ask and look.

The night before the surgery, I said goodbye to Thomas. I told him how much I loved him. He cried for the first time about my condition. Matt and I tried to sleep, but the rest didn't come.

In the early morning of March 30—Good Friday—I changed into a hospital gown, surgical cap, and mask. A routine EKG was run. It took several tries before they could get the IVs in. The attempts were painful and caused extra bruising.

I said goodbye to my mom and Matt and was wheeled into the Cath lab, this time alone.

The three- to four-hour surgery stretched longer than expected. Scarred wires needed careful removal. Every tug risked tearing a vessel.

When I awoke, I was in agony. The aches were worse than before. Something new had emerged too: strange, rhythmic twitches in my abdomen. I mentioned it to the medical team, and we all assumed it was nerves firing. Still, it didn't feel natural and didn't subside.

Recovery was grueling at home. A massive hematoma swelled at the site. The veins in my arms were occluded with clots, causing intense pain. The headaches and twitching remained persistent.

My parents, Matt, and friends helped with everything—meals, Thomas, and daily tasks. Button-up shirts became my go-to. Even drying my hair felt impossible. The surgical site itched like crazy. The painful swelling in my chest radiated from the trauma.

At a follow-up interrogation with Dr. Prager, we finally uncovered the source of the strange pulses. An old failsafe epicardial wire— implanted by Dr. Miller back in 2007—now connected my ICD to the outer layer of my heart through the abdomen. Because of my low BMI, I periodically felt pulses from the electrical transmissions. They were harmless but constant, unexpected reminders of my condition. The pulsing would be something I would have to learn to live with unless I opted to have another surgery. Each day brought multiple unsettling disturbances. I quickly realized that deep breaths and adjusting my position typically caused the annoyance to disengage.

Still, I healed.

A week after the procedure, I felt up for a short hike. It was a small step toward normalcy. While out, I received news from Chief McGee that Captain Jim Spell, my confidant, and lifesaver, had succumbed to his cancer.

While I was saddened, it wasn't unexpected. I took it with relative ease, hoping that this would be the last of such losses.

Three weeks later, after a trip to the Dominican Republic, the sun and ocean worked their magic. My headaches faded, the pain subsided, and only the pulses remained.

And somehow, I felt stronger than ever.

On the day of Thomas's third-grade play, I got the call. My mom confirmed what I already anticipated: "Gammy went to be with Jesus."

She had passed peacefully that morning. I returned to the trail. At the bench where I often sat, hummingbirds buzzed above me. Then, high above, an eagle soared.

If God allows the departed to send signs, I saw them in those wings—Gammy and Papa T—together again, hovering close.

But Gammy always said, "Life can change in an instant."

As I descended the trail, I found a friend standing over a man in distress. She asked me to stay while she went for help.

The man collapsed beside me. "My body is failing," he said.

Fearing the worst, "I'm so sorry." I told him. "It's part of life. We all fail eventually." I mentioned Gammy's passing that morning. "She's in heaven now."

His eyes flickered. "Today?"

I nodded.

I didn't know if this man had another day or another ten years, but at that moment, I hoped he had something to believe in. As we waited, I thought of Gammy's spirit. She had always believed in carrying on, no matter what life threw at her.

When paramedics arrived, I said a silent prayer of thanks—for him, for Gammy, for life.

At Gammy's funeral, her ninety-nine-year-old sister stood hunched, but still standing. Her loved ones surrounded her open casket, an old tradition from the family business. Thomas and his cousins peered in close. I hung back. The moment felt peaceful, not heavy.

They laid her to rest beside Papa T and her stillborn baby Wright. Watching the coffin lowered made me reflect on my close call in 2007.

If I had died back then, that's likely how they would have buried me, six feet under.

I thought about how I really preferred cremation—ashes scattered in the mountains I love.

Gammy lived a whole life seeking perfection, and now, in heaven, she finally found it.

As I trudged the trail again, I reached into my pocket and released a pinch of paper confetti—each piece a memory of Doug, Steve, Jim, and Gammy. These people were gone, and nothing was going to bring them back. The only thing I could do was acknowledge and appreciate the time we had.

With a prayer, I whispered my gratitude and released the paper.

"Lord, thank you for the days spent with these souls—for their love, encouragement, and the legacy they leave.

Wherever they are—by your side, in another life, or woven into the mystery—may they feel my love and yours.

For in the end, beneath it all, what remains is our love."

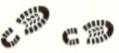

STEP TO REDUCE ANXIETY AND INCREASE HEART HOPE:

Prepare for what's beyond. Knowing the trail ends gives deeper meaning to the adventure.

Conclusion

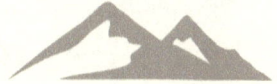

Looking back, I see now that every experience—even the darkest, most painful ones—served a purpose greater than myself. Without the storms, I might never have noticed the light. Without the unseen hand that saved me, I would have been dead and gone, crushed beneath my despair.

I often wonder: how did I get through it all? The truth is, you get up each day, take what comes, and respond as your heart is led. And sometimes—just being—is the best you can do.

There's no perfect formula for surviving the days of your life. You keep moving, step by step, trusting that somehow, it all matters.

I've already outlived the average survival by a decade, and if it's within the will for my life, I intend to live another twenty years. Nearly two decades have passed since that defining moment, and while I've come a long way, I'd be lying if I said I had it all figured out.

My brain, permanently affected by a lack of oxygen, still faces cognitive hurdles. Thinking on the spot is difficult, and words don't always come easily. I've stood before large audiences with prepared remarks, only to blank without my notes. In everyday conversation, I often mix up names or use the wrong words—not from distraction, but because my mind is working overtime to keep up.

These struggles have deepened my natural introversion. I rehearse conversations in my head, anticipate topics, document names—anything to feel more prepared. I stay quiet, not out of disinterest, but because I'm trying to speak with care. And sometimes, that effort means saying nothing at all.

People often wonder what dying from cardiac arrest feels like—to have your heart suddenly stop. Aside from a flash of dizziness, there's no pain. No fear. It's a quiet, unexpected release. It's the kind of passing we should all hope for.

I still see cases of cardiac arrest misreported, with only modest improvements in survival. Yet, awareness is growing.

Last year in Rosemary Beach, Florida, I noticed several defibrillators placed at the public edge of private boardwalks—a tactic still relatively rare. I couldn't help but wonder if the highly visible AEDs we had installed throughout the Vail Valley over ten years prior had inspired others to bring the idea home.

Personally, I've made peace with my body—most days—but the pressures never entirely go away.

Living in this world, as humans, is a battle. But I've come to believe this: it's not the physical that defines you. It's what's rooted deep in your soul.

I'll likely live the rest of my life with an ICD or some form of implanted equipment guarding my heart. The scars, pulses, shocks, procedures, and complications are reminders of what survival costs. One day, when the rest of my body fails, the device will be turned off so my soul can move on.

It's a small price to pay for the gift of more time.

The anxious, spiraling thoughts may never fully disappear, but I've learned to manage them—with the practices and hope I've shared throughout these pages.

My heart literally stopped once. And in that moment, everything became clear: life is fragile, fleeting, and far too precious to spend chasing someone else's definition of enough.

Cardiac arrest forced me to face how temporary many of our pursuits truly are. We give ourselves to things that will never sustain us. That's why we must draw the line in our hearts—protecting us from the forces we allow to define us. True satisfaction doesn't come from meeting every standard. It comes from embracing what's real. What's lasting.

Just yesterday, a neighborhood friend who organized a CPR training for her pickleball group called to tell me that one participant used the skills to save a life in California. One small seed planted long ago bloomed far beyond what I could have imagined.

We don't always get to see the difference we make. But we must believe every moment matters.

Each time I hear of a person who was saved because of my influence, it hits me in a way that's hard to explain. It's never just a statistic or a success story—it's a soul. A life. And in a deeply spiritual sense, I think of those lives as the children I chose. It's a truth that is tender, painful, and beautiful. It doesn't erase the ache of the children I never had. But it redeems it.

My near-death experience wasn't just a physical rupture. It was a spiritual reckoning.

I live now for something greater. Something eternal. Something real.

The questions I've carried—about life, death, and what lies beyond—couldn't fit into every chapter. That's why I included a separate added bonus: a spiritual reflection that goes deeper into the thoughts that shaped me as a survivor. It's for anyone seeking peace, purpose, or meaning. I hope it speaks to your soul.

But if this is where our journey ends, let this be what you take with you:

The trek is never easy. And yes, it ends the same for us all.

But the good news? Death is not the end.

Life—in its fullest, truest, most enduring form—begins in eternity.

Until that day, the world will keep trying to pull you in different directions. It will offer illusions, distractions, and quick fixes. But you have the power to choose something more.

You can choose love—whenever, wherever, and however it's needed. That's how we endure. That's how we overcome. Love. And that . . . is the heart of the matter.

17 Steps to Reduce Anxiety and Increase Heart Hope:

1. **Get outside and move.** Sunshine, fresh air, and motion shift your mindset and bring clarity.
2. **Don't expect easy.** Even dark seasons hold meaning and shape what's to come.
3. **Find ways to serve.** By helping others, you'll find unexpected joy and renewed purpose.
4. **Do things differently.** What once worked may no longer be the solution.
5. **Build structure.** Success happens through small, consistent actions and the support of others.
6. **Coincidences are signs.** Notice and follow the quiet directions.
7. **Ask for help.** Life isn't meant to be done alone; people want to support you.
8. **Consider your perspective.** Focusing on what you do have calms the mind and lifts the heart.
9. **Savor the good.** Reflect on the blessings in your life and what it took to receive them.
10. **Expect pain and heartache.** Acceptance is the first step toward healing and future happiness.
11. **Be honest with loved ones.** Authenticity deepens connection and builds trust.
12. **Share your story.** Your truth may be the encouragement someone else needs.
13. **Let go.** Releasing what you thought was best makes space for what is best.
14. **Honor each day.** Appreciate its purpose and time in the scheme of life.
15. **Don't stop believing.** Hope gets you through, even in the lowest moments.
16. **Build your identity on timeless principles.** It is impossible to maintain the standards of an everchanging world.
17. **Prepare for what's beyond.** Knowing the trail ends gives deeper meaning to the adventure.

References

p. 5, Grateful Dead. Live at Fillmore East, September 20, 1970. New York City, NY, 1970. Garcia, Jerry, and Robert Hunter. "Brokedown Palace." Track 6 on American Beauty. Warner Bros. Records, 1970. Grateful Dead. *The Complete Annotated Grateful Dead Lyrics*. Edited by David Dodd. New York: Simon & Schuster, 2005.

p. 40, Piper, Don, and Cecil Murphey. *90 Minutes in Heaven: A True Story of Death and Life*. Grand Rapids, MI: Revell, 2004.

p. 109, Eisenberg, Mickey S. *Resuscitate!: How Your Community Can Improve Survival from Sudden Cardiac Arrest*. 1st ed. Seattle: University of Washington Press, 2009.

p. 133, Spurgeon, Charles H. "A Lesson from the Life of King Asa." In *The Metropolitan Tabernacle Pulpit Sermons*, vol. 29, sermon no. 1732. London: Passmore & Alabaster, 1883.

Acknowledgements

Everyone wants to write a book, but few see it through to completion. Now I know why. It's difficult—and it requires tremendous support from others.

Foremost, you are reading this because of the God who controls the universe and authors all our lives. I never could have imagined—let alone orchestrated—the circumstances and extraordinary people who brought this story to life. Thank you, Lord, for saving me—even when I didn't know I needed saving. Thank you for the experiences that made it all possible.

To the most amazing human I've ever encountered—my husband, Matt. "Thank you" will never be enough. From the moment our eyes locked, you've loved me with rare, unending depth. You stood by me through my cardiac arrest, recovery, and everything that followed. You became my night nurse, my caretaker, my protector, partner, and provider. And you gave me the freedom and unconditional love I needed to heal, follow my heart, and ultimately write this book.

I know my dedication to these passion projects has, at times, felt all-consuming—even selfish. I'm sorry for the moments my activities pulled me away from you. Every action was always to fulfill my purpose in saving the lives and souls of others. Thank you for standing by me, always. I will always love you more than words can tell.

With all my love, SBPC

To my family and friends—thank you for enduring my quirks, loving me through my antics, and carrying me through life.

To Sue Froeschle and the first responders who saved me—I will forever be grateful for your selfless service and lifesaving actions.

To those who believed in Starting Hearts and supported the mission—your encouragement gave me the courage to keep going.

And to my coaches, editors, and first readers—thank you for helping me shape this narrative. Your insights and honest feedback helped transform a tangled, wordy diary into the most meaningful book I could write.

From the bottom of my heart, thank you to every person who joined me on this path. You've helped me turn pain into purpose and survival into something far greater: life.

Bonus Material:
The Big Questions

Reader Advisory: This additional content is not for everyone. Only read it if you're open to exploring big questions—and extreme possibilities. Please don't let this bonus section influence your *Heart of the Matter* review. This narrative stands alone—for seekers, skeptics, and fellow survivors on a spiritual journey. This content is also available to download on my website, **HeartHope.org.**

Answers to Life's Biggest Questions from the Perspective of a Survivor

In the nearly two decades since surviving cardiac arrest, the impermanence of life has been a constant undercurrent in my thoughts, awakening a deep curiosity about humanity's enduring mysteries. It's nearly impossible to have a brush with death and not confront life's biggest and often unanswerable questions. The philosophical inquiries we all wrestle with—Who are we? Why are we here? What happens when we die? Does God exist? Are our souls eternal?—are universal, connecting us across generations, cultures, and belief systems.

The pursuit of understanding is not confined to the walls of academia, laboratories, or the minds of survivors. It is intricately woven into our daily decisions, doubts, and dreams. Rooted in wonder, philosophy seeks explanation of disorder and clarity within the unknown.

Albert Einstein once stated that humans know less than one thousandth of one percent of all there is to know. To put that in perspective, it's like reading three letters from my book and thinking you understand the whole story. Recognizing our limitations inspires both humility and curiosity. What lies beyond that thousandth of a percent? The mysteries of matter, energy, time, and consciousness remain largely out of reach, challenging the boundaries of human understanding while also inspiring deeper exploration.

Yet, the goal of knowledge is not always to answer, but to propose, interpret, and imagine the 99.99 percent that we don't know. This spirit of inquiry has accompanied me on long walks through mountain trails, where thoughts interlace with footsteps and nature's effortless existence becomes a sanctuary for contemplation. I appreciate that many people, burdened by the pace of life, may not have the space to reflect deeply on such matters. This realization compelled me to share my insights—not as definitive answers, but as offerings born from lived experience and thoughtful observation.

Before sharing these thoughts, I turned to my two most trusted spiritual mentors—my mom and Pastor Craig. As expected, they challenged my musings, and I appreciate that. Their commitment to a strict biblical interpretation helps keep me grounded when my creativity wanders. Still, imagination is a vital part of spiritual seeking. Therefore, I share these reflections with caution, not as verity but as possibility. The truth is, once we reach the other side, everything we considered foundational here may seem inaccurate in the face of ultimate reality.

Purpose and Time of the Heart

Since surviving cardiac arrest, these subjects have taken on new intensity. Life and death are no longer abstract concepts. They are personal. Tangible. Felt.

The heartbeat, once a silent background rhythm, now occupies the forefront of my awareness. I notice its every flutter, every skip, every surge. What once went unquestioned—an automatic, invisible function—has become the focal point of my existence. I live in rhythm with it, trusting it will continue, while knowing all too well that one day, it won't.

The heart is the first organ to form in the womb and the last to quit upon death. Its job seems simple: to pump blood, to keep us alive. But its significance runs far deeper. From the very beginning, the heart tracks the time we spend on earth—each beat a marker, each pulse a countdown to its end. It sustains not only our bodies, but our presence in this world.

In contemplating the heart, I was intrigued and amazed by its universality. Every breathing creature possesses one. From the rapid flutter of a hummingbird to the slow, majestic thump of a whale, the heartbeat is a shared language—an invisible thread connecting all life. Its electrical current propels us forward, powered by forces beyond our comprehension. Just as waves crash upon the shore and the sun rises and sets without our command, the heart moves to an unseen cadence.

Science tells us the heart is powered by electricity—an impulse. But where does that impulse originate? Who or what commands it to begin and allows it to cease?

The more I pondered, the more reverence I felt. The heart is both mechanical and mysterious, biological and divine. It is the physical engine of life—and perhaps the spiritual one as well. In many traditions, the heart is not only the source of life, but the seat of the soul.

Still, the human heart is not eternal. No matter how strong or persistent, it will one day fall silent. And when it does, we are left to wonder: *What happens when it's over?*

Surviving a near-death experience demands a reckoning with this reality. Death is not just probable—it's certain. One hundred percent of everything that lives dies. And though we fear the moment our hearts stop beating, what we really fear is what lies beyond. The unknown. The separation from all we know and love. But death, like birth, is part of a design—a transition, not an end.

Man has always attempted to make sense of it. Some envision a paradise. Others, a return to the earth. Though the visions differ, most converge on a shared longing of continuation. A belief that something—some essence, some spirit—lives on.

I share that belief.

I believe there is a Creator who sustains life and determines its end. A power that commands the heart's rhythm and loves the soul.

The heart is more than a pump. It charts our time and holds the spirit.

I survived cardiac arrest not just because my heart restarted—but because something willed the electrical current to continue. Something greater than medicine. Greater than chance.

In the end, the heartbeat is more than a biological rhythm. It is a quiet miracle. A sacred drum of life and time. And while I don't have the answers, I am convinced: The heart's purpose is to stop.

Who is God?

The phrase "Oh my God!" is one of the most commonly used expressions today, often uttered without thought to the profound power it may provoke. Once reserved for moments of reverence, it has become a reflexive reaction to the trivial. This raises a thought-provoking question: To whom are we speaking?

I was raised in a Bible-centered household where my mother emphasized the sacredness of God's name. Misusing it was not only discouraged but also punished—occasionally with a bar of soap. For her, reverence wasn't a tradition; it was a practice of respect, discipline, and faith.

Today, the genuine search for God often takes a backseat in a world filled with distractions. With religion fading from classrooms, media, and many households, exploring the divine can feel inaccessible or even irrelevant. But dismissing the question doesn't quiet the soul's longing to understand.

For most of my life, I accepted what I had been taught about God with little scrutiny. But my cardiac arrest was a powerful collision that pushed me to question everything—starting with whether God existed, and if so, what that meant for me and the world.

One sticking point in my "belief" was the exclusivity sometimes promoted in Christianity—that all other perspectives on God are invalid. That narrow view felt discordant with the vastness of the universe and the diversity of human experience. After facing death and reflecting on my own spiritual encounters, I rejected this rigidity.

Instead, I embraced the awe and wonder that led me to study and consider the rich demonstrations of global religious traditions. I found that while each perspective offers its unique lens, many share timeless wisdom and the yearning to connect with something greater.

I value the legitimacy of each person's interpretation. Just as every life story is unique, so too is each encounter with the righteous. My experience has not turned me away from God, but expanded my understanding of who God is—and deepened my respect for the many ways people connect with the source of life.

As someone who finds joy in simplifying complexities, I set out to distill these varied perspectives. Through interviews and research, I explored how people interpret the meaning of life, death, and God, and summarized the insights for reflection.

This chart is not exhaustive, but a starting point—an invitation to ponder how humans from all walks of life and belief systems define truth, hope, and belonging.

The table outlines foundational beliefs of major world religions and spiritual philosophies. While it does not delve into specific denominations, this is intentional. The goal is clarity and focus on the common resources that bind these perspectives. I hope this information helps you evaluate and define your beliefs.

Lynn's Side-by-Side Comparison of Spiritual Perspectives

Category	Judaism	Christianity
Beliefs	Emphasizes one supreme God as Creator and orchestrator of life; belief in a coming Messiah to save man exists. Believes the Jewish people are chosen by God for responsibility and His favor.	Affirms the one Jewish God revealed through the Trinity, with Jesus as the fulfilled Messiah and divine Son bringing salvation through death, resurrection, and eternal life.
Symbol	Star of David	Cross
Timeline	Beginning of time, documented ~1200 BCE	1st century CE, evolved from Judaism
God/Leader	Yahweh is the one and only creator, sustainer, all-knowing, eternal, indivisible God. He is merciful and has a covenantal relationship with Israel.	One God in three persons. The Trinity is: Yahweh-our Father in Heaven, Jesus-fully God and fully human, Holy Spirit-God in our hearts.
Foundational Texts	Tanakh (Torah core section), historical and prophetic scripture about God, creation and righteous living. Talmud includes Mishnah and Gemara, central for interpreting Jewish law and practice.	Bible-Old Testament-overlaps Jewish Tanakh, and New Testament-personal and historical accounts of Jesus' life, teachings and salvation.
Core Teachings	God is the giver of life, obey His covenant, laws, community	Jesus is God in human flesh, represents divine love, salvation and grace
Practices/Rituals	Prayer, kosher, tithe, synagogue services	Prayer, sacraments, tithe, church worship
Origin of Life	Created by God	Created by God
Afterlife	Souls transition to eternal afterlife united with God, or returned for spiritual growth.	Believing souls transition to eternity with a loving God in heavenly peace while waiting for God to establish the full completion of His kingdom both in heaven and earth. Unbelieving souls transition to separation and suffering.
Meaning of Life	Honor and fulfill God's laws, pursue justice, holiness and acknowledge God	Love and serve God and others, live like Jesus, and develop a personal relationship with God to be reconciled
Moral Code	Justice, kindness to strangers, charity, justice, follow commandments	Golden Rule: Love, humility, mercy, peacemaking, forgiveness, follow Ten Commandments
Est. Population	15 million	2.3 billion
Geographical Distribution	Israel, U.S., scattered globally	Global, especially Americas and Europe
Days of Worship	Shabbat (Friday evening to Saturday evening), songs, study, prayer and community at synagogue	Sunday (most denominations), songs, study, prayer and community at church
Holidays	Passover (liberation), Yom Kippur (repentance), Rosh Hashanah (new year), Hanukkah (lights)	Christmas (virgin birth of Jesus), Good Friday (death of Jesus), Easter (resurrection of Jesus)

This chart reflects my interpretation, compiled from countless online resources, personal conversations, and scholarly insights. Because the information is a synthesis of many sources, a single reference cannot be cited. It is not intended to be exhaustive or fully inclusive of all religious sects, but rather a broad snapshot of shared values and recurring themes across major spiritual traditions, serving as an introduction to understanding core beliefs.

An exploration of what humanity believes about life, purpose, death, and the divine.

Category	Hinduism	Islam
Beliefs	Teaches Brahman is the ultimate reality, an eternal, infinite, and unchanging essence; manifests in many deities. All life is sacred, yet not all Hindus stress "creator."	Stresses absolute monotheism (tawhid); Allah is the sole creator, sustainer, and judge. Muhammad is his final prophet guiding humanity.
Symbol	🕉 Sacred Vibration	☪ Crescent Moon
Timeline	Beginning of time, documented ~1500 BCE	7th century CE
God/Leader	Brahman is ultimaate reality, a formless, infinite divine essence. Deities manifest in expressions like Vishnu, Shiva, Devi.	Allah is one, unique, all-merciful, without partners. Rejects the Trinity and mortal depictions of God.
Foundational Texts	Historical and mythological scriptures: Vedas, Upanishads, Bhagavad Gita, Ramayana, and Mahabharata; texts guide philosophy, rituals, ethics, and cosmological understanding.	Quran the word of God as revealed through the Prophet Muhammad. Teachings of the prophet Hadith essential for Islamic law. Sunnah reflects Prophet Muhammad's practices and shapes Islamic daily guidance.
Core Teachings	Life is sacred and interconnected, Karma (action), Dharma (duty), and Moksha (liberation)	Submission to Allah, Five Pillars
Practices/Rituals	Worship, meditation, fasting, pilgrimage	Prayer, fasting, charity, pilgrimage
Origin of Life	Emerged from Brahman, no definitive beginning or end	Created by Allah
Afterlife	The soul is divine and eternal, reincarnated until it achieves liberation and oneness with Brahman.	The soul is eternal and faces peace and comfort for the righteous and regret and pain for the wicked.
Meaning of Life	To realize the divine within and its unity with Brahman, achieve liberation from suffering	Submit to and worship Allah, be obedient and express gratitude, attain closeness to God
Moral Code	Practice truth, nonviolence, compassion, self-control, and spiritual discipline	Sharia law, Five Pillars of Islam, worship, devotion
Est. Population	1.2 billion	1.9 billion
Geographical Distribution	Primarily South Asia, growing globally	Middle East, North Africa, Asia, global
Days of Worship	Daily, worship through prayers, song and meditation at shrines or temples	Prayer 5x per day, Friday (Jumu'ah) sermon and prayer at mosque
Holidays	Diwali (lights), Holi (colors)	Ramadan (month of fasting, reflection, and deep devotion), Eid al-Adha (sacrifice of Abraham)

The chart is available for download at HeartHope.org

Lynn's Side-by-Side Comparison of Spiritual Perspectives

Category	Agnosticism	Atheism
Beliefs	Holds the position that divine existence is unknowable; it is a position on knowledge, not necessarily disbelief or belief. A choice to not seek or acknowledge a deity.	Not an organized religion. The absence of belief in deities or supernatural beings. It does not prescribe morality, spirituality, or worldview.
Symbol	? Question mark	Scientific symbols
Timeline	18th–19th centuries	Ancient to modern eras
God/Leader	Uncertain about existence of God(s). Strong agnosticism believes always unknowable and weak agnosticism believes currently unknown.	Affirms no deity exists. It is a philosophical stance, not a religion.
Foundational Texts	No specific texts. Emphasis on philosophical works questioning knowledge of God, often influenced by Hume, Kant, and modern skeptics.	No specific texts. Reliance on philosophy, science, and secular writings (e.g., Dawkins, Hitchens) shape atheistic worldviews.
Core Teachings	Skepticism	Evidence-based worldview
Practices/Rituals	Questioning, exploring, openness	Ethics, logic, rational thought
Origin of Life	Unknown	Explained through science
Afterlife	Uncertain	None
Meaning of Life	Unknown	Create personal meaning
Moral Code	Philosophical ethics, questioning	Secular ethics, reason, empathy
Est. Population	500M–1B	500M–1B
Geographical Distribution	Worldwide, secular societies	Worldwide, secular regions
Days of Worship	None	None
Holidays	Non specific (may celebrate cultural or secular holidays based on personal choice)	None (secular celebrations like Earth Day or Human Rights Day are observed by some)

This chart reflects my interpretation, compiled from countless online resources, personal conversations, and scholarly insights. Because the information is a synthesis of many sources, a single reference cannot be cited. It is not intended to be exhaustive or fully inclusive of all religious sects, but rather a broad snapshot of shared values and recurring themes across major spiritual traditions, serving as an introduction to understanding core beliefs.

An exploration of what humanity believes about life, purpose, death, and the divine.

Category	Buddhism	Paganism/New Age	Sun Worship
Beliefs	Non-theistic, follows Buddha's teachings in Four Noble Truths and Eightfold Path toward enlightenment (nirvana), transcending suffering and attachment. Not centered on creator or deity.	Paganism emphasizes nature reverence, polytheism, and rituals. New Age stresses spiritual energy, healing, and cosmic interconnectedness, not singular "universal intelligence."	Views the sun as divine, sustaining life, guiding tim and symbolizing cosmic ord not simply "over mankind
Symbol	🎡 Wheel of Dharma	A radiant light or spiral	☀ Sun
Timeline	5th–6th century BCE	Ancient to modern eras	Earliest civilizations (e.g. Egypt, Inca, Aztec)
God/Leader	Not centered on creation or a supernatural being. Buddha is an enlightened teacher, not a deity. Buddha is a guide and enlightened teacher (honored, not worshipped).	Emphasizes nature-based spirituality, multiple deities, and universal energy. Diverse practices: Wicca, Druidry, New Age mysticism differ significantly.	Many sun deities exist (Ra Inti, Helios). Polytheistic I nature and regional variatio exist.
Foundational Texts	Tripitaka, Pali Canon in Theravada, Mahayana Sutras, Buddha's teachings and individual enlightenment vary widely.	Many scientific texts and mythological texts including The Bible, Wiccan Book of Shadows, Thelema, Celtic myths, astrology guides, blends ancient and modern spiritual sources.	Oral traditions, inscription solar hymns and some ritu texts from ancient Egypt, In and Vedic influence.
Core Teachings	Enlightenment, karma, rebirth	All life is interconnected	Sun as the giver of life, pow and divinity
Practices/Rituals	Meditation, mindfulness, ethical living	Meditation, energy healing, affirmation	Rituals, sacrifices, sun ceremonies
Origin of Life	Cycle of rebirth	Scientifically, it emerged	Sun as the source of creati
Afterlife	Reincarnation or state of nirvana.	Transition to other realms or dimensions, and reincarnation.	Varies; often reincarnation merging with the divine
Meaning of Life	End suffering, achieve Nirvana	a journey of soul evolution	Harmony with nature, honoring the sun
Moral Code	Eightfold Path, ahimsa (non-harming)	Do no harm, align with universal law	Respect for nature, ritua offerings
Est. Population	500 million	1 billion	Historical, remnants in cultural practices
Geographical Distribution	Primarily Asia, global reach	Worldwide	Ancient civilizations worldw
Days of Worship	Varies, often daily meditation at shrine or temple	None	Dawn or times aligned wit sun rituals, nature
Holidays	Vesak (Buddha's birthday)	Flexible and personal, traditional holidays (Christmas, Easter) reinterpreted symbolically	Solstices (winter and summer), Equinoxes, and other solar festivals

The chart is available for download at HeartHope.org

Despite varying narratives, the question of God remains one of the most compelling. For many, God is a personal being, a creator and sustainer, the embodiment of love and justice.

I don't know the origin of God, but I do know something more powerful than myself exists—a presence that transcends explanation. Whether through the wonder of a star-filled sky or the quiet assurance that life has meaning, I sense magnificence woven into existence.

No single tradition has all the answers. But each offers a fragment of truth, an invitation to deeper connection and contemplation.

It is plausible that the many ancient accounts and spiritual traditions are different interpretations of the same universal source— distorted over time like a primitive game of telephone, but still all pointing to the one Creator.

After a long and sincere exploration, I found peace in entrusting my life to a singular, all-powerful God. This led me away from mythologies shaped by human imagination and toward belief systems grounded in historical depth and personal experience.

Of all these, I found the God of the Judeo-Christian tradition to be most compelling.

This God claims eternal existence and offers grace to all. He is described as the beginning and end, the light in darkness, the breath of life, and the source of love itself. He requires no grand rituals, only a heartfelt acknowledgment.

Honestly, the truest way to reduce anxiety and find hope for your heart is to trust in the Highest Power. When you release control to something greater than yourself, repose naturally follows.

If you've never opened your heart to the idea of something bigger than your life, what holds you back?

Belief could be your pathway to peace—in this life and the next. If that belief proves unfounded, you lose nothing. But if it is true, the reward is incomprehensible: purpose within struggle, peace amid suffering, and the promise of eternity with God and those we cherish.

In the end, my search for truth and understanding brought me back to an expanded view of Christianity. It's here I've found peace:

in the belief that God's love extends to *all* for eternity, and comfort for the pains of earth is found through trust in the teachings of Jesus Christ, the Messiah—the God of Heaven revealed in human form.

The fact is, Jesus didn't come on behalf of religion or the Bible; He came to speak of God and serve as His example—to reveal love and free mankind from the burdens of legalism and sin. Religion is humanity's attempt to quantify and interpret God's presence.

Our spiritual beliefs are often seen as dividing walls. Yet, most theological systems don't encourage judgment or division. At their core, most faith traditions emphasize peace and righteous living. A better world begins when our common truths bind us together instead of driving us apart. Rather than seeking unity through opposition, we should seek harmony in the values we share.

If God is truly the Creator of the heavens and the earth, His essence must be universal—transcending any single interpretation. To connect with such a boundless being, we must resist the temptation to reduce such power to our limited perceptions.

The greatest challenge with embracing inclusivity of all perspectives isn't the act itself—it's the absence of a single foundation to turn to when life becomes unclear.

The Book of Revelation declares that "every tribe and tongue" will worship before God. If that's true, who am I to judge the language or expression of someone else's soul? Whether through ritual or silence, temples or churches, whispers or written word—perhaps it's all the same voice, calling us home.

I am convicted that God's mercy extends beyond human boundaries. Spiritual journeys rarely follow level ground, but there is common ground in our collective surrender and shared yearning for meaning. By embracing love—the message at the heart of all sacred teachings—we find unity.

Ultimately, the question, *Who is God?* may never be fully answered. But the search for that answer—through reflection, learning, and dialogue—enriches our lives. We've mastered systems to navigate life under the sun, yet in our self-reliance, we often forget our deep need for something greater—something eternal.

God is the Creator of the universe, the sustainer of life, and the mystery that invites us to explore. While we may never fully grasp God's existence, the journey itself draws us closer.

This is why I share what I've learned—not to dictate beliefs, but to encourage others to ask, *Who* is God? In the asking, we discover life's purpose.

Where Do God and our Eternal Souls Reside?

The words spoken by God in John 8, "I am the light of the world," echoed through me as I traced the sun's glow, wondering if this was the closest physical representation of divinity I would ever know. I thought back to all my prayers—times I closed my eyes tightly and waited for a feeling, a whisper, a sign. But what if it was right in front of me the whole time—blazing, brilliant, and undeniable? The sun isn't God, of course. I'm not suggesting God is the sun, as Moses warned against worshiping celestial bodies, emphasizing that God transcends physical forms and is not confined to any one place. But the sun is a powerful parallel—the center of our existence, reigning in the heavens, high above and unattainable. It is an ever-present fire at the core of our universe. The giver of all light, the sustainer of life. Its radiance neither wavers nor fails; an ancient force that demands both reverence and fear. The sun is the regulator of time, the measure of our days, the marker of seasons. It is both comforter and provider, an omniscient existence with the singular power to see all, scorch all, nourish all, illuminate all, and comfort all. Every living thing turns toward it instinctively, worshiping in silent praise. The sun reigns and rules over all, and all the earth revolves around it. Without it, there is no life. And I couldn't help but wonder: could God reside in something so grand and so nearby? Maybe He wasn't as distant as I had once thought. Maybe every sunrise is an invitation to remember, to look upward, to acknowledge Him.

This idea led me to ponder the eternal nature of the human soul. While astrology has long linked celestial bodies to earthly affairs, I believe stars could represent more than cosmic markers—they may be spiritual vessels, illuminating the heavens with eternal radiance. There's something about the stars that calls to every soul—something sacred and everlasting. On quiet nights, when the sky stretches endlessly above, I feel as though I'm looking into a realm beyond time and human understanding.

The idea that heaven, our eternal destination, exists in the heavens, where souls shine like stars, aligns with the timeless imagery in Scripture. God speaks of people as lights in a dark world, comparing them to stars that pierce the night sky. Believers are promised to shine like stars forever—a powerful truth that suggests our spirits endure, continuing to influence, illuminate, and be known. God also says He created and knows the stars by name—and likewise, He knows His people at the time of their creation. This personal connection between the Creator and His celestial beings has always intrigued me. If He names them, watches them, cherishes them—could they be more than just burning orbs? Could they reflect what we become?

To me, this connection is more than a metaphor—it is a divine lateral. A possibility that our spirits may transcend physical life and take their place among the stars. The book of Revelation even describes stars falling to earth, shaken from the heavens. Could this be symbolic of souls returning—restored, resurrected? Even the fall of Satan is told through star imagery—cast down from glory, his soul likened to a fallen star. If rebellion leads to that descent, maybe faithfulness preserves believers in their heavenly place until the miraculous return.

Still, I acknowledge the mystery. The truth of where our eternal souls reside is not something we can fully comprehend. And perhaps we're not meant to. Faith itself is a journey through the unknown—a choice to trust in what we cannot yet see.

I find peace in believing that our spirits do not fade but endure—guiding, watching, whispering through the night.

In that boundless sky, there is the lingering consideration: If heaven exists, what about hell? It's a question most wrestle with: How could a loving God condemn anything to eternal punishment?

Before rectifying this concept, I'd like to clarify, the Bible references "hell" sparingly, and most mentions portray it not as a physical location but as a state of spiritual separation from God.

To make sense of perdition, I've considered two possibilities. First, what if hell isn't a fiery underworld, but something more familiar—our present reality, stripped of spiritual connection? The "eternal suffering" may be symbolic of a diminished existence on earth. Perhaps, in rejecting God in this life, the soul returns not as a human being capable of choice, but as a lower life form—driven by instinct, lacking freedom. I think of the Devil, cursed to slither on the ground. Could this be more corresponding imagery? Might condemned souls return as animals subject to survival's grind, stripped of voice and spirit, existing beneath man's foot and forced to abide by the sun's light? Still, this is only a theory—speculative, without certainty.

The second idea is more hopeful: universal salvation. The Book of Philippians says, "every knee will bow, every tongue confesses." If that's true, perhaps all souls will, eventually, acknowledge God—and be reconciled. Maybe, in time, every spirit finds its way home. I want this to be true. It comforts me.

But I recognize the danger of leaning on unconfirmed hopes, such as animalistic reincarnation or universal salvation. The most significant risk is that eternity isn't assured, and secondly, it eliminates the joy and peace available both in this life and in the future.

If these questions stir your heart, I encourage you: read historical books. And more importantly, ask God—if He exists—to speak to you.

I don't have all the answers. But I know this: guaranteeing eternal life isn't found in speculation. It's found in the hearts that seek it.

Preparing for the Inevitable

Every trail has a destination. Every traveler must prepare for the end.

Ironically, death is life's only certainty—yet few of us prepare. The heart can only carry the soul so far.

To walk unprepared is to risk leaving questions unanswered, peace unfound, and our true destination unknown.

Preparing for death is not surrendering to fear—it's embracing purpose. It's our spirit's responsibility.

To walk—and finish—well:

1. **Reflect on Beliefs**: Take time to explore your spiritual views. Study historical faith traditions and teachings. Let them shape your understanding.
2. **Decide in Your Heart**: Embrace the certainty of death. Choose your core convictions and let them guide your life.
3. **Live What You Believe**: Align your actions with your faith. Through love, service, and intention, let your life reflect your values.

Like a fork in the trail, we must choose. The time to decide isn't later—it's now, while the path is still ahead.

Crises like my near-death experience reveal what truly matters. For me, that moment awakened trust, gratitude, and purpose.

We will never find certainty—but we can have faith. In surrendering to that mystery, we find peace.

So ask yourself: *What do I believe?* When the time comes, who will you call on?

The trail awaits your answer. Walk it with purpose—and let your heart lead the way.

About the Author

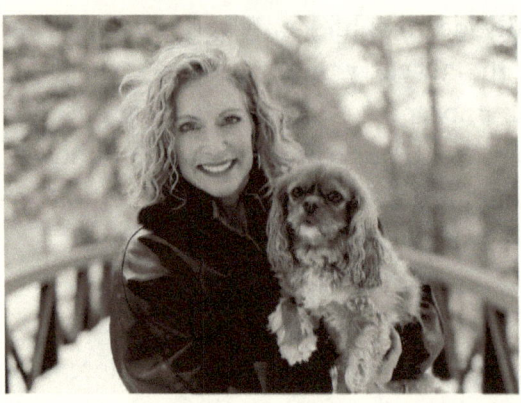

Lynn Blake is a survivor, advocate, and leader in the movement to save lives from sudden cardiac arrest. In 2007, at just twenty-seven years old, she survived a near-death experience thanks to the immediate use of CPR and a defibrillator—an experience that changed the trajectory of her life. Determined to transform her survival into purpose, she has devoted herself to raising awareness, improving survival rates, and advancing public health initiatives.

Her advocacy has sparked international awareness campaigns, legislative advancements, and earned recognition from organizations such as the American Heart Association and the American Red Cross.

Outside her work, Lynn is a devoted wife and mother who finds joy and peace in the mountains of Colorado. Whether hiking, skiing, or reflecting on the beauty of nature, she draws strength and inspiration from the people and world around her.